Mariya Doneva

Compressed Sensing for MRI

Mariya Doneva

Compressed Sensing for MRI

Advances in the sampling, sparsifying transforms, and reconstruction methods

Südwestdeutscher Verlag für Hochschulschriften

Impressum/Imprint (nur für Deutschland/only for Germany)
Bibliografische Information der Deutschen Nationalbibliothek: Die Deutsche Nationalbibliothek verzeichnet diese Publikation in der Deutschen Nationalbibliografie; detaillierte bibliografische Daten sind im Internet über http://dnb.d-nb.de abrufbar.
Alle in diesem Buch genannten Marken und Produktnamen unterliegen warenzeichen-, marken- oder patentrechtlichem Schutz bzw. sind Warenzeichen oder eingetragene Warenzeichen der jeweiligen Inhaber. Die Wiedergabe von Marken, Produktnamen, Gebrauchsnamen, Handelsnamen, Warenbezeichnungen u.s.w. in diesem Werk berechtigt auch ohne besondere Kennzeichnung nicht zu der Annahme, dass solche Namen im Sinne der Warenzeichen- und Markenschutzgesetzgebung als frei zu betrachten wären und daher von jedermann benutzt werden dürften.

Verlag: Südwestdeutscher Verlag für Hochschulschriften GmbH & Co. KG
Dudweiler Landstr. 99, 66123 Saarbrücken, Deutschland
Telefon +49 681 37 20 271-1, Telefax +49 681 37 20 271-0
Email: info@svh-verlag.de

Zugl.: Lübeck, Universität zu Lübeck, Diss., 2010

Herstellung in Deutschland:
Schaltungsdienst Lange o.H.G., Berlin
Books on Demand GmbH, Norderstedt
Reha GmbH, Saarbrücken
Amazon Distribution GmbH, Leipzig
ISBN: 978-3-8381-1101-8

Imprint (only for USA, GB)
Bibliographic information published by the Deutsche Nationalbibliothek: The Deutsche Nationalbibliothek lists this publication in the Deutsche Nationalbibliografie; detailed bibliographic data are available in the Internet at http://dnb.d-nb.de.
Any brand names and product names mentioned in this book are subject to trademark, brand or patent protection and are trademarks or registered trademarks of their respective holders. The use of brand names, product names, common names, trade names, product descriptions etc. even without a particular marking in this works is in no way to be construed to mean that such names may be regarded as unrestricted in respect of trademark and brand protection legislation and could thus be used by anyone.

Publisher: Südwestdeutscher Verlag für Hochschulschriften GmbH & Co. KG
Dudweiler Landstr. 99, 66123 Saarbrücken, Germany
Phone +49 681 37 20 271-1, Fax +49 681 37 20 271-0
Email: info@svh-verlag.de

Printed in the U.S.A.
Printed in the U.K. by (see last page)
ISBN: 978-3-8381-1101-8

Abstract

Magnetic resonance imaging (MRI) is a non-invasive imaging modality, which offers high spatial resolution and excellent soft tissue contrast without employing ionizing radiation. MRI is sensitive to a wide range of contrast mechanisms that allow assessment of both morphology and physiology, making it a modality of choice for many clinical applications.

A major limitation of MRI is that data acquisition is relatively slow, which besides being unpleasant for the patient, can also seriously degrade the image quality. Modern MR scanners are already operating at the point where further improvements in data acquisition speed by means of hardware and pulse sequence design are constrained by physical and physiological limitations. With the advent of parallel imaging techniques, this problem has partially been addressed. However, further reduction of imaging time is desired, making the development of methods which allow image reconstruction from reduced amount of data necessary.

Recently, a new sampling theory under the name compressed sensing (CS) has emerged, suggesting that image reconstruction from reduced amount of data can be achieved by exploiting the signal sparsity. The ability to reconstruct images from small number of measurements provides a new method to accelerate the data acquisition in MRI. Initial studies have shown that compressed sensing has a great potential to improve the imaging speed in MRI.

This work explores and extends the concept of applying compressed sensing to MRI. A successful CS reconstruction requires incoherent measurements, signal sparsity, and a nonlinear sparsity promoting reconstruction. To optimize the performance of CS, the acquisition, the sparsifying transform and the reconstruction have to be adapted to the application of interest. This work presents new approaches for sampling, signal sparsity and reconstruction, which are applied to three important applications: dynamic MR imaging, MR parameter mapping and chemical-shift based water-fat separation.

A radial data acquisition scheme based on the golden ratio is explored as a potential practical sampling approach for dynamic CS-MRI. This acquisition scheme provides incoherent sampling with undersampling in all spatial dimensions. It is of special interest in dynamic imaging because it allows a lot of freedom in choosing the size and the position of the time frames. No a priory planning of the dynamic scan is required and the sampling scheme is appropriate for both periodic and non-periodic dynamic applications.

A very sparse signal representation can be obtained if the sparsifying transform is adapted to the signal of interest. In this work, a method for designing a sparsifying transform, based on the knowledge of a signal model, describing the data in MR parameter mapping is presented, which achieves higher sparsity compared to other commonly used transforms leading to an improved CS reconstruction.

The application of compressed sensing for accelerated chemical shift-based water-fat separation is explored, in which the water and fat images and the field inhomogeneity map are related to the corresponding k-space data by a nonlinear transform. A reconstruction method based on a nonlinear measurement model is presented, which allows integrated compressed sensing reconstruction and water-fat separation.

The methods presented in this work allow to more fully exploit the potential of compressed sensing to improve imaging speed. Future development of these methods, and combination with existing techniques for fast imaging, holds the potential to improve the diagnostic quality of existing clinical MR imaging techniques and to open up opportunities for entirely new clinical applications of MRI.

Acknowledgements

I can no other answer make, but thanks, and thanks

— WILLIAM SHAKESPEARE

It is a great pleasure to thank all the people who helped and supported me through the last few years.

I would like to express my special gratitude to Prof. Alfred Mertins, for supporting this external work. Through the years, Alfred has played an important role in my development as a scientist, giving me guidance, support and freedom in pursuing my research directions. He was the one who first gave me a reason why is it good to know how to invert matrices, who initiated my work in research, and who made me curious about compressed sensing. I am grateful to have worked with him.

This work was performed in collaboration with Philips Research Laboratories in Hamburg, Germany, where I spent most of the time for the last three years. I would like to thank the head of the Tomographic Imaging group, Dr. Dye Jensen, for giving me the opportunity to perform this work and showing so much interest in my research.

I am very much indebted to Dr. Peter Börnert, who brought me into the field of MRI and was patiently guiding me during this work. His contagious enthusiasm, commitment and invaluable support have made the work with him a great pleasure. I am grateful for the many fruitful discussions, a lot of helpful critique, but most of all I thank him for his honesty, trust and encouragement, which have pushed me to perform at my best. Peter, when I grow up I want to be more like you.

I want to thank Dr. Holger Eggers for his valuable support. I am grateful for the many helpful discussions, tips and tricks in reconstruction and for thoroughly correcting my manuscripts, including this work. Holger is one of the smartest and most precise persons I have ever met. I hope I have caught a little bit of these qualities.

I want to express my gratitude to Dr. Christian Stehning, who has been a great discussion partner and a source of inspiration in many projects. I big thank you also to Dr. Julien Senegas, Dr. Jürgen Rahmer, and Dr. Kay Nehrke, with whom I collaborated on different projects within the last years.

A special thanks also goes to Prof. John Pauly from Stanford University for the excellent iv

collaboration and the opportunity to work in his team. I have been very fortunate to work and share an office with Dr. Michael Lustig during the time at Stanford. Miki is an amazing person. His inexhaustible energy, out-of-the-box thinking, and great sense of humor have made the work with him a great experience. I am very grateful for the many discussions we had in Stanford and later during our continued collaboration. I also thank him for joining my exam committee.

Also, thanks to all my colleagues and friends at Stanford University, and especially to Will Grissom, Huan Santos, Bill Overall, Nikola Stikov, Joelle Barral, Hattie Dong, Daeho Lee, Uygar Sumbul, Emine Saritas, Tolga Cukur, Tao Zhang, for the great time spent together.

I am grateful to my office mate Alfonso Isola for the nice and quiet working environment. A big thank you also to Tobias Voigt for the nice PhD time spent together. We started almost simultaneously and shared the same fate for the last three years. The time spent on the John Malkovich floor would have never been the same also without the company of Hanno Homann, Eberhard Hansis, Ronny Ziegler and Sebastian Zander.

I am indebted to my many colleagues for providing a stimulating and fun environment in which to learn and grow. This is a good place to thank our skipper Peter Koken, the crew of the gourmet boats Peter Mazurkewitz, Stefanie, Christian, Daniel, Peter Venickel, Friederike as well as Claas, Oli, Falk, Johan, Holger, Bernhard, Dietrich and Dirk for the great time on sea. For the great time on land I also thank Ulrich, Tim, Jochen, Ingmar, Steffen and Sascha. I would like to thank Thomas Blidung, Otmar Tschendel and Heino Svensson for the IT-support and Gabi Ziem for the assistance with posters.

I would like to express my special gratitude to my friends, in particular Ginka, Erik, Dilyan, Katya, Lora, Robert, Sasho, Ani, Bela, Radko, Milena, Chris, Mura, Angel, Elena, and Zlatka for bringing joy to my life and making Hamburg feel like home.

None of what I have done would have been possible without the love and support of my family. I would like to thank my parents Nesi and Ivan for their constant support and encouragement and my little sister Gery for being a great friend. I want to thank my parents-in-law Mitka and Anton and my brother-in-law Sasho who accepted me as a part of their family.

Finally, I want to thank my husband, Ivan for his patience and support, and for loving me the way I am.

Contents

CHAPTER ONE

INTRODUCTION

Magnetic resonance imaging (MRI) is a non-invasive imaging modality based on the concept of nuclear magnetic resonance (NMR). Compared to other imaging modalities, MRI has several unique advantages, which make it preferable in many clinical applications. MRI offers high resolution and excellent soft tissue contrast without employing ionizing radiation. MRI also provides cross sectional images with arbitrary orientation as well as true three dimensional images. Unlike other modalities, MRI is sensitive to a wide range of contrast mechanisms. These allow assessment of both morphology and physiology, giving access of parameters like flow, diffusion, perfusion, blood oxygenation, and many others.

A major limitation of MRI is that data acquisition is relatively slow. A long scan time is undesirable because of patient discomfort. In addition it limits the clinical workflow and can seriously degrade the image quality as a result of variations in the imaged object during the data acquisition, for instance caused by motion or flow. Furthermore, it limits the capability to temporally resolve dynamic processes such as cardiac motion or contrast agent bolus in angiography.

Since MRI was first introduced in the early 1970s, imaging speed has been improved dramatically. This has mainly been achieved by improvements in hardware and pulse sequence design to achieve faster data acquisition. Modern MR scanners are already operating at the point where further improvement in data acquisition speed is limited by physical and physiological limitations. However, in many clinical applications imaging speed is still a limiting factor. An improvement in imaging speed might significantly improve the quality and accuracy of clinical diagnosis.

Further improvements in imaging speed can be achieved by reducing the amount of acquired data, required to perform image reconstruction without degrading image quality. A recent development in MRI with significant impact in improving imaging speed is parallel imaging, which applies simultaneous data acquisition with an array of independent RF coil elements. The spatially variable reception sensitivities of the individual coil elements provide an additional signal encoding mechanism which allows image reconstruction with reduced number of measurements.

Other methods for scan acceleration using reduced data sampling rely on redundancies in the MR images. The associated reconstruction methods require some prior knowledge about the image. Methods in this class include partial Fourier imaging, which exploits the conjugate symmetry of k-space, and methods exploiting the spatio-temporal correlations in dynamic imaging.

In 2004, a new sampling theory coined compressed sensing emerged, suggesting that signal reconstruction from reduced amount of data can be achieved by exploiting signal sparsity. The main idea of compressed sensing is to acquire data in an efficient way, such that the number of measurements is directly proportional to the signal's information content. In the special case of MR imaging this implies that if an MR image is compressible, which is to some degree true for all MR images, data acquisition can be performed in a way that image compression is performed already within the acquisition process. In compressed sensing (CS), the data are acquired as a small set of incoherent measurements. The image is then obtained by applying a nonlinear sparsity promoting reconstruction. The ability to reconstruct images from reduced amount of data and thus accelerate the acquisition has attracted a lot of interest in the MR community, leading to active research in this area.

This work explores and extends the concept of applying compressed sensing in MRI. A very sparse description of compressed sensing given in just three keywords would be: Acquisition, Sparsity, and Reconstruction. These three aspects refer to the following questions, which arise whenever applying CS: How to acquire the data? How to find a good sparse signal representation? How to reconstruct the image? Unfortunately, there is no single answer to each of these questions that gives an optimal solution for all cases. Instead, to optimize the performance of CS, the acquisition, the sparsifying transform, and the reconstruction have to be adapted to the application of interest.

The present work considers these three aspects and presents methods for the adaptation of the CS principles to different applications.

Non-Cartesian data acquisition based on radial trajectories is investigated as a practical sampling pattern for compressed sensing, which allows undersampling in all spatial dimensions. Golden ratio profile ordering is applied to obtain incoherent and nearly uniform sampling. This sampling pattern is of special interest in dynamic imaging, because it provides a lot of freedom in choosing the size and the position of the time frame, which can also be done retrospectively.

Signals are often sparse in some transform domain. However, finding the optimal sparsifying transform for a given signal requires some prior knowledge. In this work, a method for designing a sparsifying transform is presented, which is based on the knowledge of a model describing the data in MR parameter mapping. The model-based sparsifying transform achieves higher sparsity compared to other commonly used transforms and leads to improved CS reconstruction.

Compressed sensing is based on the assumption of a set of linear measurements. However, in some applications, the image of interest is related to the measurements by a nonlinear transform. Therefore, the application of CS for accelerated chemical shift based water-fat separation is explored, in which the measurements are considered as a nonlinear transform, which maps the water and fat images and the field inhomogeneity map to the corresponding k-space data.

The outline of this book is as follows:

Chapter 2 provides a brief introduction to conventional MR imaging. It introduces the principles of signal formation, data acquisition and image reconstruction in MRI, necessary for understanding the MR part of the work. The theoretical background of compressed sensing and considerations of its application to fast MR imaging are presented in Chapter 3. This chapter describes the basic implementation of CS in MRI and gives a short overview of the state of the art in CS-MRI. In Chapter 4 an incoherent non-Cartesian sampling based on the golden ratio is explored as a potential practical sampling pattern in CS-MRI. Examples for dynamic cardiac imaging and hand imaging are presented. Chapter 5 presents a method for designing a sparsifying transform based on a known data model. The method is considered for the application of MR parameter estimation, in particular T_1 and T_2 mapping. Chapter 6 considers the application of CS for water-fat separation and presents a reconstruction method based on a nonlinear measurement model. Finally, Chapter 7 contains a summary of the work presented in this book as well as a discussion of possible future research directions.

CHAPTER TWO

PRINCIPLES OF MRI

The list of potentially workable generalized Fourier methods could go on indefinitely; there are an infinite number of ways to scan the k domain which will successfully place into the FIDs sufficient information to permit image formation from the FIDs. Each of these encoding schemes will have advantages and disadvantages in terms of quality of image information it conveys, and in terms of ease of implementation of its gradient program, and its sampling and decoding (computational) procedures. Some of these unrealized methods appear to offer significant performance advantages.

— DONALD TWIEG

This chapter discusses the image formation principles of MRI. The main focus is on the signals, on what they are, and on how are they generated and detected. The image formation process is viewed as a linear system, the notion of k-space is introduced, discussing the limitations and flexibility of k-space sampling.

2.1 Nuclear Magnetic Resonance

Magnetic resonance imaging (MRI) relies on the quantum mechanical phenomenon of Nuclear Magnetic Resonance (NMR). In clinical MRI, most commonly hydrogen nuclei (protons) are imaged, because of their high natural abundance in the human body.

The spin of an atomic nucleus can be characterized by its quantum number, which for protons is $\frac{1}{2}$. The relationship between the spin and the magnetic moment $\boldsymbol{\mu}$ that arises from it can be described as:

$$\boldsymbol{\mu} = \gamma \mathbf{S}, \tag{2.1}$$

where $\gamma = e/2m$ is the gyromagnetic ratio of the considered atomic nuclei ($\gamma/2\pi = 42.57$ MHz/T for protons in water), and $\mathbf{S}$ is the spin angular momentum.

Under the influence of an external magnetic field B_0 the magnetic moments of the atomic nuclei with spin $\frac{1}{2}$ can orient either parallel or anti parallel to the magnetic field. For a nucleus with spin $\frac{1}{2}$ these orientations correspond to two distinct energy levels

$$E_\pm = \pm \frac{\gamma \hbar B_0}{2}, \tag{2.2}$$

where $\hbar$ is the Planck constant.

If electromagnetic radiation is applied to the aligned spins with an energy equal to the energetic difference between the two states, or $E = \gamma \hbar B_0$, a transition between the two energy levels occurs. The characteristic resonance frequency of this transition is known as the Larmor frequency:

$$\nu = \frac{\omega}{2\pi} = \frac{E}{h} = \frac{\gamma}{2\pi} B_0. \tag{2.3}$$

This resonance frequency can also be thought of as the frequency at which the spins precess around the axis of the magnetic field B_0. As seen in the equation above, the Larmor frequency is directly proportional to the magnetic field strength, and is specific to a given nucleus. The Larmor frequency of the same type of nucleus also varies in different chemical compounds. These variations are due to variations in the electron distribution in chemical species, which cause slightly different magnetic shielding resulting in differences in the local magnetic field. The relative difference in the resonance frequency of one species to a reference resonance frequency is called chemical shift

$$\delta = \frac{\nu - \nu_{ref}}{\nu_{ref}}. \tag{2.4}$$

As an example, the chemical shift between hydrogen nuclei in water and in fat is about 3.35 ppm.

Since the energy difference between the two energy states is small relative to the thermal energy at room temperature, the probability of the nuclear spins occupying either orientation is nearly identical. However, there is a slight excess of nuclear spins (few ppm) with parallel alignment, which corresponds to lower potential energy. This small imbalance produces net magnetization (the volume average over the magnetic moments of the spin system) in the direction of the external magnetic field, governed by the Boltzmann statistics, which is given by:

$$\mathbf{M} = M_0 \mathbf{z} = \frac{\gamma^2 \hbar^2}{4 k_B T} B_0 \rho \mathbf{z}, \tag{2.5}$$

where k_B is the Boltzmann constant and T is the temperature in Kelvin, and the unit vector $\mathbf{z}$ gives the direction of the external magnetic field. The spin density ρ is a characteristic of the object being imaged and depends on its chemical content and structure.

The magnetization vector, as a macroscopic entity, can be tilted away from the $\mathbf{z}$-direction by applying a radio-frequency (RF) excitation pulse (i.e. B_1 field) of the appropriate resonance frequency orthogonal to the **z** direction:

$$\mathbf{B}_1(t) = \begin{bmatrix} B_{1x}(t) \\ B_{1y}(t) \\ 0 \end{bmatrix} \tag{2.6}$$

The application of the RF pulse results in time varying magnetization in the transverse plane $(\mathbf{x} - \mathbf{y})$. This phenomenon is described by the Bloch equation.

$$\frac{d\mathbf{M}}{dt} = \gamma\left(\mathbf{M} \times \mathbf{B}\right), \tag{2.7}$$

where **B** is the total magnetic field. Equation (2.7) is a general form of the equation of motion of the spin system that describes the precession of the net magnetization vector about the **z** axis. Important corrections arise from the interactions of spins with their surroundings, processes which are referred to as relaxation phenomena. The Bloch equation describes a left screw rotation about **B** with angular velocity given by the Larmor frequency ω so that the angular velocity vector is pointing in the negative **z** direction.

$$\boldsymbol{\omega} = -\omega\mathbf{z} \tag{2.8}$$

The overall effect of the RF pulse is characterized by the flip angle α, by which the equilibrium magnetization is rotated out of the **z** direction, according to the Bloch equation (2.7).

$$\alpha = \gamma \int_0^\tau |B_1(t)|dt \tag{2.9}$$

The magnetization vector immediately after an RF pulse with flip angle α is:

$$M_z = M_0 \cos(\alpha)$$
$$M_x = M_0 \sin(\alpha) \cos(-\omega t)$$
$$M_y = M_0 \sin(\alpha) \sin(-\omega t) \tag{2.10}$$

The transverse component of **M** is often written as a single complex value $\mathbf{M}_{xy}$.

$$\mathbf{M}_{xy} = M_0 \sin(\alpha) e^{-i\omega t} = \hat{M}_{xy} e^{-i\omega t} \tag{2.11}$$

2.2   Relaxation

After the RF pulse has been turned off, the magnetization vector starts to return back to the direction of the static magnetic field. It is most advantageous to analyze the magnetization and its differential equations in terms of parallel and perpendicular components. For the case of non-interacting spins, the corresponding components of the cross product in the Bloch equation lead to two decoupled equations.

$$\frac{dM_z}{dt} = 0 \tag{2.12}$$

and

$$\frac{d\mathbf{M}_{xy}}{dt} = \gamma \mathbf{M}_{xy} \times \mathbf{B}, \tag{2.13}$$

where

$$\mathbf{B} = \begin{bmatrix} 0 \\ 0 \\ B_0 \end{bmatrix}. \tag{2.14}$$

The modeling of the spin interactions with their neighborhood leads to additional terms in equations (2.12) and (2.13) which depend on decay parameters, that are different in the two equations. This difference is related to the fact that, in contrast to a given magnetic moment, the magnitude of the macroscopic magnetization is not fixed, since it is a vector sum of many spins. The components of $\mathbf{M}$ parallel and perpendicular to the external magnetic field relax differently in the approach to their equilibrium values.

The magnetic moments will tend to line up parallel to the external magnetic field in order to reach their minimum energy state. Since the spins are considered to be in thermal contact with the lattice of nearby atoms, the thermal interactions between the spins and the lattice present a mechanism for energy transfer allowing the longitudinal magnetization to return to its equilibrium state. The rate of change of the longitudinal magnetization dM_z/dt is proportional to the difference $M_0 - M_z$. The proportionality constant is empirically determined and represents the inverse time scale of the growth rate.

$$\frac{dM_z}{dt} = \frac{1}{T_1}(M_0 - M_z), \tag{2.15}$$

where T_1 is the experimental 'spin-lattice relaxation time'. The relaxation of the longitudinal magnetization from $M_z(0)$ immediately after the RF pulse to the equilibrium value M_0 is described by the equation:

$$M_z(t) = M_z(0)e^{-t/T_1} + M_0(1 - e^{-t/T_1}) \tag{2.16}$$

Spins experience local fields, which are combinations of the applied field and the fields of their neighbors. Since variations in the local field lead to different local precession frequencies, the individual spins tend to lose coherence in time, reducing the net magnetization vector. The total transverse magnetization is the vector sum of all the individual transverse components. This process is characterized by another empirical value, the spin-spin relaxation time T_2. The differential equation (2.13) is extended by the addition of the decay rate term

$$\frac{d\mathbf{M}_{xy}}{dt} = \gamma \mathbf{M}_{xy} \times \mathbf{B} - \frac{1}{T_2}\mathbf{M}_{xy} \tag{2.17}$$

The additional term leads to an exponential decay of the magnitude of the transverse magnetization.

$$\hat{M}_{xy}(t) = \hat{M}_{xy}(0)e^{-t/T_2} \tag{2.18}$$

Considering the relaxation processes described above, the final expressions for the net magnetization after an α RF pulse become:

$$M_z(t) = M_0 \cos(\alpha)e^{-t/T_1} + M_0(1 - e^{-t/T_1}) \tag{2.19}$$

$$M_{xy}(t) = M_0 \sin(\alpha)e^{-t/T_2}e^{-i\omega t} = \hat{M}_{xy}(t)e^{-i\omega t} \tag{2.20}$$

2.3   Signal detection, spatial encoding, and k-space

If a receive coil is placed near the object, the oscillating magnetization vector induces a voltage in the coil. This voltage is the MR signal that is used for imaging. The complex MR signal, thus measured, is the volume integral of the transverse magnetization in the entire object.

$$s(t) = \int C(\mathbf{r})M_{xy}(\mathbf{r}, t)d\mathbf{r} \tag{2.21}$$

$$= \int C(\mathbf{r})\hat{M}_{xy}(\mathbf{r}, t)e^{-i\omega(\mathbf{r})t}d\mathbf{r} \tag{2.22}$$

Here, $C(\mathbf{r})$ represents the RF coil reception sensitivity, which depends on the particular geometry of the coil and its position relative to the imaged object. Inserting equation (2.20) in (2.22), the following expression is obtained for the received signal:

$$\begin{aligned} s(t) &= \int C(\mathbf{r})M_0(\mathbf{r})\sin(\alpha(\mathbf{r}))e^{-t/T_2}e^{-i\omega(\mathbf{r})t}d\mathbf{r} \\ &= \frac{\gamma^2\hbar^2}{4k_BT}\int C(\mathbf{r})\sin(\alpha(\mathbf{r}))B(\mathbf{r})\hat{\rho}(\mathbf{r})e^{-i\omega(\mathbf{r})t}d\mathbf{r} \end{aligned} \tag{2.23}$$

Here, $\hat{\rho}$ denotes the signal density (extended spin density), which represents the spin density weighted by factors reflecting relaxation processes. The aim of MR image reconstruction is to obtain the signal density $\hat{\rho}$ at every point of the imaged object. Except for $\hat{\rho}$, all other three spatially dependent functions in equation (2.23) are known or measurable and can (in principle) be used for spatial encoding at different imaging stages. In the most general case the spatial encoding function may be defined as:

$$E(\mathbf{r}, t) = \frac{\gamma^2\hbar^2}{4k_BT}C(\mathbf{r})\sin(\alpha(\mathbf{r}))B(\mathbf{r})e^{-i\omega(\mathbf{r})t} \tag{2.24}$$

Thus, equation (2.23) can be simplified to:

$$s(t) = \int E(\mathbf{r},t)\hat{\rho}(\mathbf{r})d\mathbf{r}$$
$$= \langle E(\mathbf{r},t), \hat{\rho}(\mathbf{r}) \rangle \tag{2.25}$$

The measured signal can be interpreted as inner product between the encoding function and the signal density. The signal $s(t)$ and the encoding function $E(\mathbf{r},t)$ are measured at discrete times t_n. The signal density is reconstructed at discrete space positions $\mathbf{r}_n$. The signal density, reconstructed at these discrete positions is also known as the voxel signal, since ideally it is the signal which will be represented in the volume element $\Delta V = \Delta x \Delta y \Delta z$ at position $\mathbf{r} = (x,y,z)$. In the case of two dimensional imaging, it is called the pixel signal.

$$\hat{\rho} = \hat{\rho}(\mathbf{r}_n) \tag{2.26}$$

The discretized form of equation (2.25) is:

$$\mathbf{s} = \begin{bmatrix} s_1 \\ s_2 \\ \vdots \\ s_N \end{bmatrix} = \begin{bmatrix} \langle E_1(\mathbf{r}_n), \hat{\rho}(\mathbf{r}_n) \rangle \\ \langle E_2(\mathbf{r}_n), \hat{\rho}(\mathbf{r}_n) \rangle \\ \vdots \\ \langle E_N(\mathbf{r}_n), \hat{\rho}(\mathbf{r}_n) \rangle \end{bmatrix} \tag{2.27}$$

Here, the i-th row of the encoding matrix E represents the values of the encoding function at time t_i evaluated at the discrete space positions $\mathbf{r}$.

$$E_{m,n} = E_m(\mathbf{r}_n) \tag{2.28}$$

Writing equation (2.27) in compact matrix notation leads to:

$$\mathbf{s} = \mathbf{E}\hat{\boldsymbol{\rho}} \tag{2.29}$$

Equation (2.29) represents a generalized reconstruction problem, where the entries of the encoding matrix $\mathbf{E}$ depend on the particular image acquisition technique.

2.3.1   Gradient encoding

In conventional MRI, spatial encoding is achieved by applying spatially varying magnetic fields on top of the static magnetic field $B_0(\mathbf{r})$. A spatially uniform RF excitation field is applied to rotate the magnetization vector by a flip angle $\alpha(\mathbf{r}) = \alpha_0$. A receive coil, which exhibits a spatially homogeneous receive sensitivity, is used and the MR signal, detected according to equation (2.22), is simplified to:

$$s(t) = \int \hat{\rho}(\mathbf{r}) \exp^{-i\omega(\mathbf{r})t} d\mathbf{r} \tag{2.30}$$

where the resulting constant factors are also included in the signal density $\hat{\rho}(\mathbf{r})$.

The spatially varying magnetic field $B(\mathbf{r})$ is generated by applying magnetic field gradients in all three directions $\mathbf{G} = (G_x, G_y, G_z)$. The magnetic field gradients are given by:

$$G_x = \frac{dB_z}{dx} \tag{2.31}$$

$$G_y = \frac{dB_z}{dy} \tag{2.32}$$

$$G_z = \frac{dB_z}{dz} \tag{2.33}$$

Here the static magnetic field is applied in the $\mathbf{z}$ direction. In the presence of the magnetic field gradient $\mathbf{G}$ the local magnetic field is given by:

$$B(\mathbf{r}) = B_0 + \mathbf{Gr} \tag{2.34}$$

Three different types of spatial encoding are commonly used in MRI: slice selection, phase encoding and frequency encoding.

Slice Selection. Magnetic resonance occurs only in a subvolume, where the RF pulse matches the Larmor frequency. If a gradient in z direction $B = B_0 + G_z z$ is applied during an RF excitation pulse with single frequency ω, only a thin slice is selected at:

$$z = \frac{\omega - \gamma B_0}{\gamma G_z} \tag{2.35}$$

After the excitation pulse the detectable transverse magnetization in the sample is essentially a two dimensional distribution.

Phase Encoding. If a gradient field in the y direction is applied for a given time interval τ, the Larmor frequency will vary in this direction during that time interval, so that the signal at different positions accumulates a different phase. After the gradient has been switched off, the precession frequency returns to a constant value over the plane, while the imprinted phase remains proportional to y. This process is called phase encoding.

$$\phi(x, y) = (\omega(x, y) - \omega_0(x, y))\tau = \gamma G_y y \tau \tag{2.36}$$

Frequency Encoding. If a constant gradient G_x is applied to the sample, the frequency of precession will change linearly with location, too.

$$\omega(x, y) = \gamma G_x x \tag{2.37}$$

If the signal is read out while this gradient is on, contributions from different locations along the x axis will exhibit different frequencies. This process is called frequency encoding, and the corresponding gradient is called frequency encoding gradient, also sometimes referred to as read gradient.

2.3.2 K-space

For a general gradient $\mathbf{G}$, the phase accumulated in the received MR signal at time t after the beginning of the gradient is given by:

$$\phi(\mathbf{r}, t) = \gamma \int_0^t \mathbf{G}(\tau)\mathbf{r}d\tau \tag{2.38}$$

Using the following definition the k-space coordinate can be given as:

$$\mathbf{k}(t) = \gamma \int_0^t \mathbf{G}(\tau)d\tau \tag{2.39}$$

and the induced signal (2.30) now reads:

$$s(\mathbf{k}) \quad = \quad \int \hat{\rho}(\mathbf{r})e^{-i\mathbf{kr}}d\mathbf{r}. \tag{2.40}$$

The vector quantity $\mathbf{k}$ defined as the integral of the gradients can also be seen as a vector of spatial frequency coordinates. The idea of employing the so called k-space to describe gradient encoding was introduced by Twieg [1, 2], and this convention greatly simplifies the concept of the time-domain signal in MRI. Using the k-space notation, the spatial encoding functions, generated by switched gradients, are given by :

$$E_k(\mathbf{r}) = e^{-i\mathbf{kr}}. \tag{2.41}$$

The spatial encoding functions in conventional imaging are Fourier basis functions, hence, this type of spatial encoding is also called Fourier encoding. Thus, the signal $s(t_n)$, sampled discretely in time, fills the Fourier space (or k-space), and an image is reconstructed according to Eq. (2.40) by applying an inverse Fourier transform to the acquired data set (Figure (2.1)).

$$\hat{\rho} = \mathbf{E}^{-1}\mathbf{s} = \mathcal{F}^{-1}(\mathbf{s}) \tag{2.42}$$

This shows the sequential manner of conventional MRI (samples in k-space are obtained at discrete times t_n) that limits the image acquisition speed. In the case of Cartesian k-space sampling, the Fast Fourier Transform (FFT) algorithm can be applied for fast reconstruction.

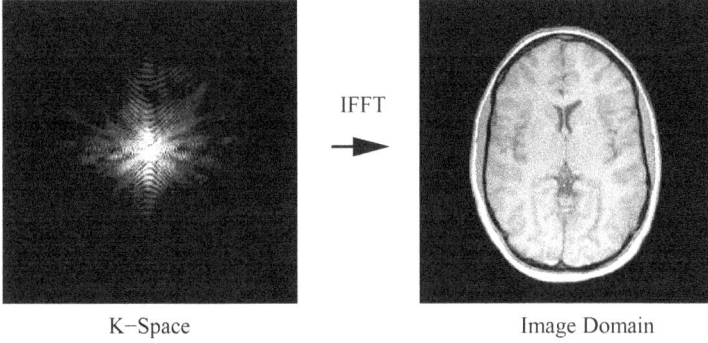

K–Space   Image Domain

Figure 2.1. Fourier Encoding. The image is reconstructed from the measured k-space data by applying a discrete inverse Fourier Transform

2.3.3 K-space traversal in 2D Cartesian MRI

This section describes how the image acquisition is performed in standard 2D Cartesian MRI. A typical gradient echo sequence is used as an example, which is schematically shown in Fig. 2.2.

An RF pulse is applied to tilt the magnetization away from the direction of the static magnetic field to the transverse **x-y** plane as described in section 2.1. To select a 2D slice within the three-dimensional object to be imaged, a constant gradient G_z is applied during the RF pulse. To rephase the spins in the slice, a reversed gradient with half of the moment is applied immediately after the pulse [3]. Next, phase encoding and read gradients have to be applied for the spatial signal encoding within the selected 2D slice. Before application of these gradients, there is no encoding in the k_x-k_y plane, which corresponds to the 2D k-space origin $k_x = k_y = 0$. Applying a gradient in the read direction causes the signal to dephase. For a constant gradient G_x this can also be seen as movement in the k_x direction of k-space.

$$k_x(t) = \gamma G_x t \qquad (2.43)$$

In Fig. 2.2 a) a negative gradient is applied to move to $-k_{x,max}$. Similarly, applying a gradient in the k_y direction corresponds to movement in k_y. The simultaneous application of these gradients leads to the diagonal traversal of k-space shown in Fig. 2.2 b). At this point in the experiment, the magnetization has been prepared, and signal acquisition can take place. During signal acquisition, a read gradient G_x is applied. this time with positive sign. This gradient causes the magnetization to rephase, or in terms of k-space moves the signal toward the center of k-space in the read direction. A complete rephasing of the spins results in magnetization echo and the continued application of the read gradient results in a further dephasing of the spins. The echo occurs at the point where the gradient moments are completely

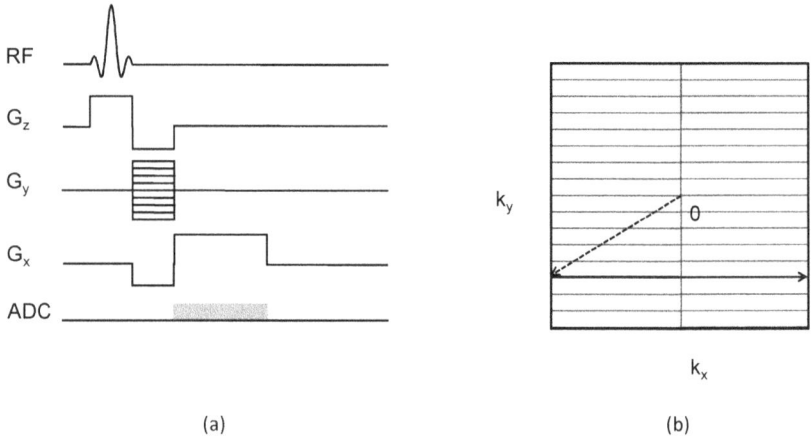

Figure 2.2. Gradient echo experiment. (a) Schematic representation of a gradient echo experiment. The top line shows the timing in the transmit channel, followed by the slice, phase, and read gradients, and the bottom is the acquisition channel. (b) Traversal of k-space for the gradient echo sequence shown in a). The k-space is filled line by line.

compensated. For a readout gradient with the same amplitude as the dephasing gradient which is applied for twice the time, the echo is in the middle of the readout line.

In the described experiment only one line of k-space is acquired. In order to obtain a full coverage of the 2D k-space, the experiment has to be performed multiple times with different step in the phase encoding. This is achieved by altering the amplitude of the phase encoding gradient each time, which is indicated with multiple lines in the phase encoding gradient in Fig. 2.2 a). For example, for a matrix size of 256×256, 256 data points have to be acquired in the read direction and 256 phase encoding steps must be performed. Denoting the time between two subsequent excitation pulses with TR (repetition time), the total time for the experiment is equal to 256 TR.

In three dimensional imaging, the whole imaging volume is excited and two phase encoding gradients and one read gradient are used for the 3D spatial encoding. For an imaging matrix of $256 \times 256 \times 256$, 256×256 phase encodings must be performed, drastically increasing the imaging time.

2.4 Restrictions and flexibility of data sampling in k-space

2.4.1 Resolution and FOV

In the case of uniform Cartesian sampling, the k-space coverage is determined by the Nyquist sampling theorem. For the case of a constant read gradient G_x such sampling is achieved along the frequency encoding direction by taking data at uniform intervals Δt in time with the k-space step

$$\Delta k = \gamma G_x \Delta t. \tag{2.44}$$

The discrete uniform sampling of k-space results in periodicity of the image space. The k-space sampling frequency determines the length of the period, or so called field of view (FOV).

$$FOV \propto \frac{1}{\Delta k} \tag{2.45}$$

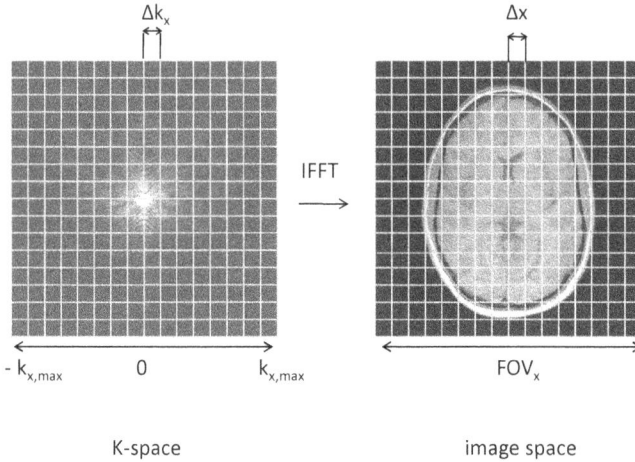

K-space   image space

Figure 2.3. Field of view and resolution in Cartesian sampling. The FOV in the image domain is proportional to the inverse of the k-space sampling interval. Denser sampling of k-space corresponds to larger FOV. If the encoded FOV is smaller than the object to be imaged, aliasing occurs. The image resolution is inversely proportional to the maximum extent of the covered k-space.

The finite sampling of k-space results in a finite resolution of the reconstructed image. The image resolution is given by the extent of the k-space sampled:

$$\Delta x \propto \frac{1}{2k_{x,max}} \tag{2.46}$$

Thus, to achieve a higher resolution, a larger area in k-space has to be covered. Increasing the k-space sampling density results in a larger FOV. If the encoded FOV is smaller than the object being imaged, the signal outside the FOV will fold back causing aliasing artifacts. Higher sampling density in the frequency encoding direction does not cost additional time. This is why oversampling in the frequency encoding direction is typically applied to prevent aliasing.

2.4.2 K-space trajectories

Cartesian k-space sampling is the most frequently used sampling pattern. One of its important advantages is that the image reconstruction is a simple Fourier transform, which is easily implemented and very efficient. Cartesian sampling is also relatively insensitive to many system imperfections. However, the acquisition of data in k-space is not limited to the rectilinear Cartesian sampling. In fact, there is considerable freedom how to acquire data in MRI. By altering the encoding gradients in an appropriate way one can achieve different trajectories to traverse the k-space. A few examples of the most popular non-Cartesian trajectories are shown in Fig. 2.4.

The most common non-Cartesian trajectory is the radial trajectory [4]. The radial, also known as projection reconstruction (PR), trajectory is advantageous because the center of k-space is often resampled during the acquisition, making such a dataset relatively robust against motion or flow artifacts [5]. Another common non-Cartesian trajectory is the spiral sampling, which exists in several different variations [6–8]. K-space is usually covered with a few interleaved spiral readouts, with longer read duration. The PROPELLER trajectory [9] is a hybrid between Cartesian and radial sampling and is advantageous because the overlapping central parts of k-space can be used for motion correction. Other sampling trajectories found in the literature are rosette [10], Lissajou [11] and stochastic [12]. Many others can be imagined.

In an ideal imaging experiment, where the subject is exactly on resonance, the gradients do exactly what they should, there is no signal relaxation, and no subject motion, all different k-space trajectories should work well and the only difference remains the image reconstruction. In practice, these conditions do not hold and the effect of these imperfections in the measured signal with different trajectories plays an important role in the quality of the resulting image. Thus, different k-space trajectories might be advantageous for different applications.

The Nyquist sampling theorem determines the sampling rate for a perfect reconstruction of a signal sampled uniformly on a Cartesian grid. For nonuniform sampling, usually the Nyquist limit is applied to the largest distance between two samples in k-space. Another generalization of the sampling theorem for non-uniform sampling states that a band-limited signal can be perfectly reconstructed from its samples if the average sampling rate satisfies the Nyquist condition [13]. Therefore, although uniformly spaced samples may result in easier reconstruc-

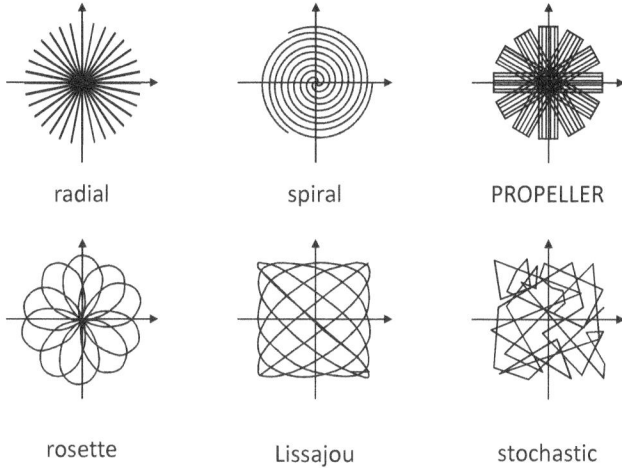

Figure 2.4. Non-Cartesian k-space trajectories.

tion algorithms, it is not a necessary condition for perfect reconstruction. Undersampling in non-Cartesian trajectories also leads to artifacts. However, these artifacts are often not as pronounced as in Cartesian sampling and in many cases could be tolerable. Specifically for trajectories with variable sampling density, such as radial, often very few artifacts are present. This is because the k-space center, where usually most of the signal energy is concentrated, is fully sampled. Radial sampling is often used with undersampling to reduce the scan time [14].

2.4.3 Gridding

One disadvantage of non-Cartesian data sampling is the difficulty of reconstructing the resulting data sets. If k-space data are acquired on a non-Cartesian grid the image reconstruction is not anymore as simple as applying an inverse FFT. To be able to use FFT, a common approach is to first resample the data to Cartesian grid points. There are several different approaches to resampling. Here the convolution gridding will be described, which is the most commonly used resampling method in nonuniformly sampled k-space MR imaging.

Gridding is the estimation of a uniformly sampled rectilinear k-space data set given the original non-uniformly sampled data (Fig. 2.5).

The gridding algorithm, adapted to MRI by O'Sullivan [15] and Jackson [16], involves convolving each non-Cartesian k-space sampling point with a dedicated convolution kernel and resampling the result to the appropriate Cartesian k-space grid locations. In variable density sampling, the k-space data are corrected for their sampling density before the interpolation.

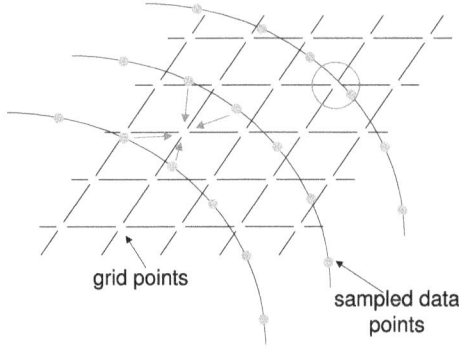

grid points

sampled data
points

Figure 2.5. Gridding. The non-uniformly sampled k-space data are interpolated to estimate the data values on a rectilinear grid

This procedure is given by equations (2.47) and (2.48)

$$M'_s(k_i) = M_s(k_i)DCF(k_i) \tag{2.47}$$
$$M''_s(k_j) = [M'_s(k_i) * C(k)] \, III(k_j). \tag{2.48}$$

The k-space data $M_s(k_i)$ measured at non-uniform sampling locations k_i is first multiplied with the density correction function $DCF(k_i)$ (Eq. (2.47)). The density corrected data $M'_s(k_i)$ is then convolved with the gridding kernel $C(k)$ and resampled on the Cartesian grid k_j, which is denoted as multiplication with the delta train $III(k_j)$. The convolution with the gridding kernel $C(k)$ in k-space leads to a multiplication of the image with $c(r)$ (the inverse Fourier transform of the kernel $C(k)$) in image space (Eq. (2.49)). While O'Sullivan et al. [15] concluded that the theoretically optimal gridding kernel is an infinite sinc function, its application in practice is computationally infeasible.

$$m''_s(r_j) = \mathcal{F}^{-1}\{M''_s(k_j)\} = m_s(r_j)c(r_j) \tag{2.49}$$
$$m_s(r_j) = m''_s(r_j)/c(r_j), \quad c(r) = \mathcal{F}^{-1}\{C(k)\} \tag{2.50}$$

Therefore, gridding kernels with compact support in k-space are used instead. This results in intensity variation (apodization) of the data in the image domain. In a post-processing step, called deapodization, the effect of the gridding kernel apodization in the spatial domain is removed by division with the inverse Fourier transformed filter kernel as given by Eq. (2.50).

When choosing a convolution function one has to consider the behavior of its inverse Fourier transform $c(r)$. First, $c(r)$ should have no zeros within the FOV, because this will cause large artifacts in the image. Second, if $c(r)$ has significant energy outside the FOV, this energy will fold back in the image. A common choice for the gridding kernel is the Kaiser-Bessel window [16], which gives a good compromise between computational complexity and reconstruction error.

2.5 SNR and imaging speed limitations

Two important limitations in MRI are the signal-to-noise ratio (SNR) and the imaging speed. These will be briefly described in this section.

2.5.1 SNR

The SNR is an important indicator of the image quality in MRI. The SNR can be defined as the signal level S divided by the standard deviation of the image noise N.

$$SNR = \frac{S}{\sigma(N)} \tag{2.51}$$

Since the signal in MRI is proportional to the applied static magnetic field one way to improve the SNR is by applying a stronger magnetic field (high field MRI). The SNR can also be improved by using an array of small surface coils placed close to the body. In a coil array, each coil element captures a strong signal from a local region and the contribution, to both signal and noise, from the rest of the sample is negligible. Thus, coil arrays have the advantage of yielding higher signal-to-noise-ratio (SNR) over a large FOV compared to whole body coils [17]. The MR signal is also inversely proportional to the temperature, however there is little we can do about the subject temperature in in vivo imaging.

Noise from a number of sources can enter into magnetic resonance data acquisitions and can affect the quality of the reconstructed images. Two principal classes of noise sources involve i) the radio-frequency (RF) coil array and associated electronics used to acquire the MR signal, and ii) the object or body being imaged. The balance of these noise sources depends on a number of conditions (e.g. the magnetic field strength, the size and number of detector coils, the performance of the preamplifier). In modern MR scanners, coil noise is usually very small compared to the noise from the imaged sample.

Besides the above mentioned noise mechanisms, the SNR can be affected by the acquisition parameters. The received noise energy is proportional to the square root of the acquisition bandwidth $\sqrt{BW} = 1/\sqrt{\Delta t_x}$ at which the signal has been sampled. Large bandwidth reduces the SNR, but allows faster imaging. The signal is proportional to the voxel size $\Delta V = \Delta x \Delta y \Delta z$. Again here, there is a trade off, this time between SNR and resolution.

A common method to improve the SNR is to use signal averaging. Repeating the experiment several times the signal intensity increases by the number of averages, whereas the noise increases by the square root of the averages, leading to improvement of the SNR at the cost of an increased acquisition time.

The SNR is a major limitation in MRI, because of the very small signals being detected. There is a connection between SNR, image resolution and acquisition time and it is generally not possible to improve the one without deteriorating one of the others. However, imaging speed is a critical factor in many applications and in the case that the SNR is high enough to accommodate such losses, possibilities for increasing the imaging speed can be examined.

2.5.2   Fast MR imaging

The total imaging time needed to form an image in MRI is given by the number of required RF excitations times the repetition time TR. In conventional MR imaging, often a single phase encoding line is acquired after each RF excitation. This means that for a 3D experiment the total acquisition time is

$$T_{acq} = N_y N_z N_a TR, \tag{2.52}$$

where N_y and N_z are the number of phase encoding steps in y and z directions and N_a is the number of averages.

From equation (2.52), it can be seen that one way to improve the imaging speed is to decrease the repetition time TR. For the gradient echo sequence shown above, the shortest TR possible is dictated by characteristics of the applied gradients. In order to shorten the minimum TR and keep the same FOV and resolution, stronger gradients have to be applied for shorter time. A lot of work has been done in the past in improving the gradient strengths and switching times, and modern MR scanners often operate at the limits of gradient strength and slew rate. Also, physiology provides a fundamental limit to gradient system performance as high gradient amplitudes and rapid switching can produce peripheral nerve stimulation [18]. This means that a further decrease in the total scan time using faster gradients is not feasible.

One can also change the way the data are acquired in order to accelerate the scan. This can be achieved by acquiring more than one phase encoding line after an RF excitation. An extreme case is single shot EPI [19], where the whole k-space is covered after a single RF excitation. Multi-echo measurements are affected by mixed contrast effects (the different k-space lines are acquired at different times and have different contrast) and signal loss due to relaxation.

Another way to improve the imaging speed is to reduce the number of phase encoding lines. This can be done by skipping the outer phase encoding lines at the cost of reduced resolution or increasing the distance between adjacent phase encoding lines, which decreases the FOV in the phase encoding direction. Reducing the FOV leads to decreased SNR and if the reduced FOV is smaller than the object to be imaged to foldover artifacts.

In parallel imaging [20–22], simultaneous data acquisition with multiple coils in a coil array is used to accomplish part of the spatial encoding traditionally performed by the gradient fields alone. This additional sensitivity encoding allows to reduce the number of phase encoding lines without reducing the FOV or image resolution. The achievable scan acceleration factor in parallel imaging depends very much on the coil array characteristics. Theoretically, if the coil array presents a set of orthogonal encoding functions, an acceleration factor equal to the number of channels can be achieved. In practice, this is difficult to achieve. Large coil arrays with up to 128 coil elements have been introduced in the past [23, 24] to boost SNR and allow higher reduction factors. Limitations of the acceleration factors using parallel imaging include on the one hand rapidly decreasing SNR with increasing acceleration factors due to numerical instabilities and on the other hand the difficulty in developing coil arrays with large numbers of elements that are well decoupled and have independent sensitivity patterns.

Finally, also prior knowledge can be used in the reconstruction to reconstruct images from reduced k-space data. Probably the simplest of these methods is partial Fourier imaging [10, 25, 26]. In partial Fourier imaging it is assumed that the image phase varies slowly over the FOV. Data acquisition is performed asymmetrically, covering a little bit more than half of k-space. The image phase is estimated from a small part of fully sampled data around the k-space origin and the conjugate symmetry of the Fourier transform is used to estimate a real-valued image.

A number of reconstruction methods rely on prior knowledge of the spatio-temporal correlations in dynamic MRI. Usually, the assumption is that the dynamic information is mainly contained in the low resolution data. In the keyhole method [27, 28] low resolution information is acquired during the dynamic scan and the high frequency information is taken from a fully sampled reference image acquired in the beginning. The RIGR method [29] applies the same sampling, however instead of replacing the high frequency information, image reconstruction is performed by fitting the measured data to a set of basis functions learned from the fully sampled reference image. In methods like k-t BLAST, k-t SENSE [30] and k-t PCA [31] also part of the high frequency information is measured and the missing data are recovered using spatio-temporal correlations learned from the low resolution data. Another reconstruction method using prior knowledge, which is particularly suited for angiography measurement is HYPR [32]. HYPR models the signal as high-resolution spatial prior (an image obtained over a longer time with no temporal information) multiplied with low-resolution dynamic information allowing to get better temporal dynamic information from a small amount of data in each time frame.

The main focus of this work is on accelerating MR measurements using compressed sensing, which will be explained in more detail in the next chapter. Compressed sensing exploits the signal sparsity to reduce the number of acquired data points and to reduce in this way the imaging time. This prior knowledge is very general and is not restricted to a certain type of images. However, the image sparsity can vary a lot for different applications and there can be different methods to invoke sparsity in the image. Also, sometimes additional prior knowledge can be applied to optimize the performance of CS for a given application.

CHAPTER THREE

COMPRESSED SENSING (IN MRI)

One should not increase, beyond what is necessary, the number of entities required to explain anything.

— OCCAM'S RAZOR: LAW OF PARSIMONY,
WILLIAM OCCAM (14TH CENTURY)

Compressed sensing (CS) is a new field which has seen enormous interest and growth in the recent past. In many applications, the signals of interest are compressible. In other words they can be represented in a much more compact form than the one in which they are usually acquired. Images and audio signals are a few of the many examples in which we are using compression on a daily basis. CS suggests that the signal compressibility can be exploited already in the data acquisition to reduce the amount of data that need to be measured in the first place. This concept has huge practical implications, in particular for applications in which the measurements are expensive, the number of sensors is limited, or the measurements are slow, as in MRI. In this chapter the principles of compressed sensing will be described and those will be considered especially for the application in fast MRI.

3.1 Introduction

Compressed sensing (CS) is an emerging area in signal processing and information theory which has recently attracted a lot of attention [33, 34]. The idea behind CS is that sparse or compressible signals can be acquired in an efficient way by applying compression already in the data acquisition process.

The Nyquist sampling theorem, also known as Whittaker-Kotelnikov-Shannon (WKS) theorem, states that a low pass signal is completely determined by a sequence of samples, obtained uniformly with the sampling rate at least twice the highest frequency contained in the signal [35]. The theorem also provides a formula for the reconstruction of the original signal (sinc-interpolation). The Nyquist sampling theorem is a sufficient condition for perfect signal recovery. However, for the class of sparse or compressible signals this condition is not necessary.

The idea of sampling below the Nyquist rate is almost as old as the Nyquist theorem itself. Another result in sampling theory published in 1967 due to Landau [36] gives a lower bound on the sampling density required for any sampling scheme (uniform or not) that allows perfect reconstruction. This lower bound is given by the support of the Fourier transform of the signal.

For signals with sparse support of the Fourier transform Landau's bound is much lower than the Nyquist limit. Laundau's bound applies to an arbitrary sampling scheme and is achievable for uniform sampling only for a very special case of multiband signals, for which there is no overlap between uniform translates of the spectral bands by multiples of a quantity smaller than the bandwidth. For all other signals irregular sampling is required. With few exceptions [37–39], methods for sub-Nyquist sampling based on Landau's limit usually exploit prior information about the spectral support. Compressed sensing is based on a similar idea, however it is generalized to sparsity in arbitrary transform domain and does not require explicit knowledge of the signal support in that domain.

In many applications such as imaging, astronomy, geophysics, and high-speed analog-to-digital conversion the signals we are interested in are often sparse in a certain basis. For example, a typical image taken with a digital camera, which has a few million pixels, can be very well described by a few tens of thousand of wavelet coefficients with almost no perceptual loss. In other words, the information content of a signal may be much smaller than suggested by its bandwidth. One can design efficient sampling or sensing schemes, which capture the useful information in a number of measurements directly proportional to the signal's information content. For sparse or compressible signals the required number of measurements is often much smaller than the Nyquist limit. These measurements are non-adaptive but need to be obey certain conditions in order to allow signal recovery. An example of sampling with provable signal recoverability conditions is random sampling, in which the measurements are performed by correlating the signal with a set of random vectors. However, other sampling schemes, such as randomized Fourier samples, are also conceivable. The signal is then reconstructed from what appears to be an incomplete set of measurements using a nonlinear sparsity promoting reconstruction.

The application of CS to MRI is one special application of CS, which has seen probably the highest growth so far. One reason for this is that CS is particularly suited for MRI. The measurements in MRI already represent linear combinations of pixels (Fourier coefficients) and the sampling of k-space is relatively flexible. Therefore, there is no need for any hardware modifications in order to perform CS data acquisition. Also, CS allows improvements of imaging speed, which is a crucial factor in MRI.

3.2   CS basics

This section gives a short overview of the existing CS theory. The goal is to sample a discrete signal $\mathbf{x}$ of length N. Without loss of generality, in the following sections the signal of interest will be described as a vector in an N dimensional space. Images can be brought in this form by concatenating all columns of the image in one vector. The general CS theory considers real signals ($\mathbf{x} \in \mathbb{R}^N$), although the extension to complex signals is straightforward. Since this work considers MR images, which are usually complex, it is assumed that all computations are performed with complex data.

3.2.1 Sampling

Linear measurements of $\mathbf{x}$ can be described as an inner product of sampling waveforms $\boldsymbol{\varphi}_m$ and $\mathbf{x}$.

$$y_m = \langle \mathbf{x}, \boldsymbol{\varphi}_m \rangle, \quad m = 1, ..., M. \tag{3.1}$$

The measurement vector $\mathbf{y}$ is given as the product of the measurement matrix $\boldsymbol{\Phi}$ and the signal $\mathbf{x}$

$$\mathbf{y} = \boldsymbol{\Phi}\mathbf{x}, \tag{3.2}$$

where the sampling waveforms are the rows of the matrix $\boldsymbol{\Phi}$. For an orthonormal matrix $\boldsymbol{\Phi}$

$$\boldsymbol{\Phi}^H \boldsymbol{\Phi} = I \tag{3.3}$$

the signal $\mathbf{x}$ can be recovered by simply applying $\boldsymbol{\Phi}^H$ to the measurement vector $\mathbf{y}$. In the case of oversampling $M > N$, where the number of measurements is larger than the signal dimension, usually the least squares method is applied to obtain a signal estimate

$$\hat{\mathbf{x}} = (\boldsymbol{\Phi}^H \boldsymbol{\Phi})^{-1} \boldsymbol{\Phi}^H \mathbf{y}. \tag{3.4}$$

Instead, CS considers the case in which only a small number of measurements are obtained $M \ll N$. In this case, Eq. (3.2) is an underdetermined linear system and in the general case does not have a unique solution. However, if the signal $\mathbf{x}$ is sparse and the measurement matrix $\boldsymbol{\Phi}$ satisfies certain conditions, CS suggests that the signal $\mathbf{x}$ can be recovered from what appears to be a highly incomplete set of measurements.

The following consideration provides an intuitive explanation why this is possible. Suppose that the signal $\mathbf{x}$ is S-sparse, that is it has only S nonzero coefficients and all the rest is zero. If the locations of the nonzero entries of $\mathbf{x}$ were known, the measurement matrix $\boldsymbol{\Phi}$ can be reduced to an $N \times S$ matrix $\boldsymbol{\Phi}_S$ by choosing only the columns corresponding to these non-zero locations. Similarly the vector $\mathbf{x}$ can be reduced to a vector $\mathbf{x}_S$, containing only the nonzero coefficients. This leads to a new system of equations

$$\mathbf{y} = \boldsymbol{\Phi}_S \mathbf{x}_S, \tag{3.5}$$

with only S unknowns. In this case $M = S$ measurements would be sufficient to recover the signal $\mathbf{x}_S$. The locations of the nonzero coefficients in the original signal are generally unknown, so this type of reconstruction is unpractical. Instead, CS suggests that the sparse signal $\mathbf{x}$ can be recovered "blind" (without knowledge of the signal support) from M linear measurements, with $S < M < N$, by finding the sparsest solution of the underdetermined problem.

3.2.2   Sparsity

The first fundamental premise in CS is the signal sparsity. Formally, a signal is said to be sparse, if it has many zero and few nonzero coefficients. Compressed sensing does not require sparsity in a particular domain. The signal of interest can be directly sparse, or it can have a sparse representation in some transform domain. A more realistic model for real signals is that the signal is compressible, which means that the vast majority of the information in the signal is contained in a few coefficients. The remaining coefficients are not exactly zero, but they are very small. For such signals CS can not obtain exact reconstruction. However, if the signal is well approximated by the taking the large coefficients only and setting the small coefficients to zero, CS gives an accurate reconstruction as well.

CS works on signals which are sparse or compressible. If such signals were rare or unusual, the fact that they can be acquired more efficiently might not be of very high relevance. But in fact, virtually all signals we might need to measure can be represented in a compact form in some domain. There is usually some pattern in the signal we want to acquire, which allows such sparse signal representation. Sparse signal representations have been extensively studied in the past and there are many different transformations that can sparsify different types of signals.

A piecewise constant image, for example, can be sparsely represented by applying a finite differences transform. This transform approximates the first derivative of the image in both directions. Real-life or medical images are rarely piecewise constant. However, in some cases (angiography) most of the signal information is contained in few large intensity changes and the finite differences transform can be useful. Transforms like the discrete cosine transform (DCT) and the wavelet transform are used in state of the art image compression [40, 41]. The raw images are transformed, quantized and then compressed by keeping only the largest coefficients. This is a standard compression approach which is used in lossy image coders like JPEG-2000 [41]. It allows to save memory for the efficient storage of images. Usually 5 to 10 fold compression can be achieved without any perceptual loss. The diversity of possible structures that can appear in an image is huge, therefore there is no single transform that will sparsely represent all types of images. However, there are many possible transforms to choose from as well as methods for designing a transform that sparsifies the signals of interest.

The domain, in which a signal is sparse or compressible, is referred to as the sparsity domain. The transform, which is used to sparsify the signal will be referred to as sparsifying transform $\boldsymbol{\Psi}$:

$$\mathbf{z} = \boldsymbol{\Psi}\mathbf{x} \tag{3.6}$$

There are three domains of interest. The sparsity domain is where the signal has a compact representation, i.e. the coefficient vector $\mathbf{z}$ is sparse. The signal of interest $\mathbf{x}$ is defined in the signal domain and the measurement vector $\mathbf{y}$ is acquired in the measurement or sampling domain. These domains and the transforms between them are illustrated in Fig. 3.1.

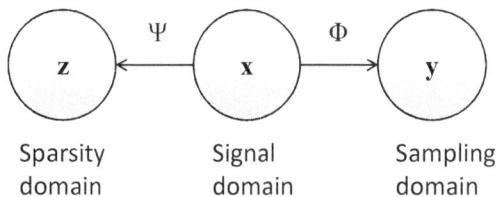

Figure 3.1. Different domains in CS. Three domains are considered in CS: the sampling or measurement domain, the signal domain which is the signal representation of interest, and the domain in which the signal has sparse representation.

Almost all the theory of compressed sensing has been developed for classes of signals that have a sparse representation in an orthonormal basis. However, for some signals there may not be any good sparsifying orthonormal basis or no good orthonormal basis is known to exist. For example, take a signal, which is a composition of two signals, the one with a sparse representation in the canonical basis and the other with sparse representation in the DCT basis (see Fig.3.2). A signal with sparse representation in the one basis is necessarily dense in the other, so the combined signal is not sparse in either basis. One can construct a so called dictionary, which is a collection of signal prototypes or so called atoms [42]. A dictionary is called overcomplete if the number of atoms is greater than the signal dimensionality. Representing the signal with respect to an overcomplete dictionary adds a lot of flexibility and significantly extends the range of applicability. The signal is represented in the form

$$\mathbf{x} = \mathbf{D}\mathbf{z} \tag{3.7}$$

where $\mathbf{D}$ is an $N \times L$ overcomplete dictionary in which there are possibly many more columns than rows.

For the example above, a dictionary can be constructed as a concatenation of the two orthonormal bases. Clearly, a sparse representation in this dictionary exists, in which each part of the signal is described by the appropriate basis. Larger dictionaries can be constructed by combining more different orthonormal bases, expanding the range of signals with sparse representation in these dictionaries. If prior knowledge about the signal exists this could be included to design an appropriate dictionary. Overcomplete dictionaries often allow much sparser signal representations than orthonormal bases. Therefore, it is natural to expect overcomplete representations to be helpful in compressed sensing problems. However, finding this sparse representation is more difficult. Since the dictionary is overcomplete, finding the signal representation is an ill posed inverse problem. The sparse representation problem is closely related

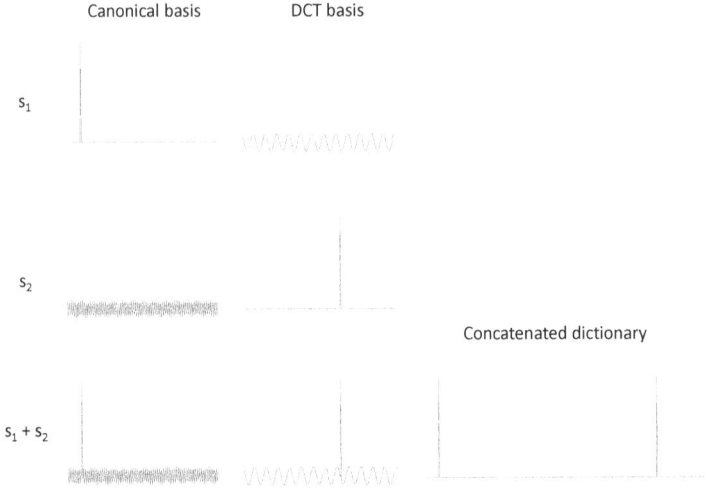

Figure 3.2. Sparsity in orthonormal bases and overcomplete dictionaries. A sparse signal in the canonical basis has a dense representation in the DCT basis and a sparse signal in the DCT basis is dense in the canonical basis. Therefore a composition of those two signals is dense in both bases. However, it can be sparsely represented in a dictionary constructed as concatenation of the two bases.

to the compressed sensing recovery problem and similar algorithms are employed for obtaining the solution.

3.2.3   Incoherence

The second premise of CS concerns the mutual coherence between the measurement and the sparsity basis. Assume that the measurement matrix $\mathbf{\Phi}$ and the sparsifying matrix $\mathbf{\Psi}$ are orthonormal bases in $\mathbb{C}^N$. Here the measurement matrix $\mathbf{\Phi}$ corresponds to the classical sampling scheme (full sampling) in time or space. The mutual coherence between the two bases is defined as the maximal inner product between the vectors of the two bases [33]:

$$\mu(\mathbf{\Phi}, \mathbf{\Psi}) = \sqrt{N} \max_{1 \leq k,j \leq N} |\langle \varphi_k, \psi_j \rangle|, \tag{3.8}$$

where the vectors φ_k and ψ_j are normalized to 1 and $\sqrt{N}$ is a normalization factor such that μ can obtain values between 1 and $\sqrt{N}$. The mutual coherence μ shows how correlated the two bases are. CS concerns pairs with low coherence. The idea of incoherence is that signals having sparse representation in a given transform domain $\mathbf{\Psi}$ must be spread out in the domain they are acquired. This allows signal recovery from a small set of samples, acquired non-adaptively in the sampling domain. The dense representation in the sampling domain means that we don't have to be careful which samples are chosen, almost any set of measurements will give a perfect reconstruction. Uniform undersampling, or measuring a set of consecutive samples are exceptions, however considering the number of all possible realizations of random sampling the probability of picking exactly these patterns is extremely low. The mutual coherence suggests a method to identify the domain in which the signal can be sparsely sampled.

Random matrices have received a lot of attention in the CS literature because they are largely incoherent with any other basis $\mathbf{\Psi}$ [33, 43–45]. Although random matrices are often used for theoretical proofs in the CS literature, their practical applicability is limited. Purely random measurement matrices are computationally inefficient, which is a limiting factor for large scale problems. Also, performing random measurements might not be trivial, and generally requires modifications in the data acquisition hardware. Fortunately, random matrices are not the only choice for data sampling in CS. The canonical basis and the Fourier basis are an example of bases pair with maximal incoherence $\mu(\mathbf{\Phi}, \mathbf{\Psi}) = 1$. Noiselets [46] are incoherent with the canonical basis, the Fourier basis and many wavelet bases.

3.2.4 Conditions for sparse signal recovery

In order to be able to recover the sparse signal from reduced number of measurements, the sampling matrix has to obey the so called Restricted Isometry Property (RIP). For signals, which are sparse in an orthonormal basis $\mathbf{\Psi}$, recovering the signal $\mathbf{x}$ is equivalent to recovering its sparse representation $\mathbf{z}$. In this case the condition is applied to the matrix $\mathbf{A} = \mathbf{\Phi}\mathbf{\Psi}^H$, which maps the sparse coefficients to the measurements. Here the measurement matrix $\mathbf{\Phi}$ is an $M \times N$ matrix and $\mathbf{\Psi}$ is an $N \times N$ orthonormal matrix.

The RIP condition was introduced by Candes and Tao [47] as a measure of quality of the sampling matrix. The restricted isometry constant δ_S is defined as the smallest quantity such that

$$(1 - \delta_S) \|\mathbf{z}\|_2^2 \leq \|\mathbf{Az}\|_2^2 \leq (1 + \delta_S) \|\mathbf{z}\|_2^2 \tag{3.9}$$

for all S-sparse signals $\mathbf{z}$. The RIP condition requires that δ_S is small. Good CS matrices have a δ_S close to 0. This prevents the sparse signal $\mathbf{z}$ being in the nullspace of the matrix $\mathbf{A}$, which assures that the signal energy is approximately preserved when applying $\mathbf{A}$ to any S-sparse vector $\mathbf{z}$. It further implies that every subset the matrix $\mathbf{A}$, containing S or fewer columns, is approximately an orthonormal matrix.

The restricted isometry constant of a matrix $\mathbf{A}$ is exceedingly hard to evaluate and essentially requires the computation of the extreme eigenvalues of all submatrices with cardinality less or equal to S. So far there is no explicit construction of matrices of any size which possess the RIP. Instead, the most successful approach has been to consider families of random matrices and determine bounds on S such that a matrix randomly drawn from the family satisfies the RIP with overwhelming probability. It is now known that many types of random measurement matrices have small restricted isometry constants [33, 43–45]. These include matrices with Gaussian or Benoulli entries as well as the matrix of randomly selected vectors of a Fourier matrix. The last example is particularly useful in MRI, since the measurements are performed in the spatial frequency domain and also because it allows fast multiplication using the FFT.

A related condition to the RIP is the so called coherence of the matrix $\mathbf{A}$. The coherence of a matrix $\mathbf{A}$ is defined as largest absolute offdiagonal entry in the Gram matrix $\mathbf{A}^T\mathbf{A}$ [48]:

$$\mu(\mathbf{A}) = \sqrt{N} \max_{j \neq k} |\langle \mathbf{a}_j, \mathbf{a}_k \rangle| \tag{3.10}$$

where $\mathbf{a}_j$ and $\mathbf{a}_k$ denote columns of $\mathbf{A}$. The matrix $\mathbf{A}$ is incoherent if μ is small. The coherence shows the similarity between the columns of $\mathbf{A}$ and is one of the few sparse-recovery metrics that can be computed for a given matrix $\mathbf{A}$ in reasonable time. Similarly to the RIP condition, low coherence ensures that the sparsest solution is unique and it could be recovered by an appropriate reconstruction algorithm. Therefore, low coherence is naturally required in CS.

All the considerations above hold for sparsity in an orthonormal basis $\boldsymbol{\Psi}$. For signals which are sparse with respect to an overcomplete dictionary the signal representation in that dictionary is generally not unique. Usually, in order to assure such unique sparse representation, the same requirements are applied as for the case of orthonormal bases. In other words, it is required that the dictionary $\mathbf{D}$ is also incoherent. Only very recently it has been shown that exact reconstruction with CS is also possible if the signal is sparse with respect to an overcomplete highly coherent dictionary.

If two columns of the matrix $\mathbf{D}$ are closely correlated, it might be impossible to distinguish between them. For example, imagine a dictionary which has two identical atoms. In this case the coherence is maximal. If a signal $\mathbf{x}$ has to be represented with respect to this dictionary, it can be explained equally good by the first or the second atom or by any combination of the two. Therefore, there is no way to reconstruct a unique sparsest solution $\mathbf{z}$ from a set of measurements $\mathbf{y} = \boldsymbol{\Phi}\mathbf{x} = \boldsymbol{\Phi}\mathbf{D}\mathbf{z}$. However, the goal is to reconstruct the signal $\mathbf{x}$ and not its sparse representation $\mathbf{z}$. If the dictionary is coherent, it is not possible to recover z, but it is still possible to recover $\mathbf{x} = \mathbf{D}\mathbf{z}$ from the measurements $\mathbf{y} = \boldsymbol{\Phi}\mathbf{x}$.

In [49], a modified RIP condition is proposed analogous to the original RIP. The restricted isometry property adapted to $\mathbf{D}$ (abbreviated D-RIP) with constant δ_S states that

$$(1 - \delta_S) \|\mathbf{v}\|_2^2 \leq \|\boldsymbol{\Phi}\mathbf{v}\|_2^2 \leq (1 + \delta_S) \|\mathbf{v}\|_2^2 \tag{3.11}$$

holds for all $\mathbf{v} \in \Sigma_S$, where Σ_S is the union of all subspaces spanned by all subsets of S columns of $\mathbf{D}$. Σ_S is just the image under $\mathbf{D}$ of all S-sparse vectors. Again, good sampling matrices have small restricted isometry constant δ_S.

The D-RIP condition is exactly as difficult to verify as the RIP condition. So far, it has been shown that certain random matrices satisfy this condition. Without being mathematically precise, one can say that in the case of CS with sparse representation with respect to overcomplete dictionaries, the measurement matrix $\mathbf{\Phi}$ needs to be incoherent, but this does not necessarily hold for the dictionary $\mathbf{D}$.

3.2.5 Reconstruction

CS suggests that the sparsest solution is the best one and it is the task of the reconstruction to find this solution. A measure of the signal sparsity is the ℓ_0 semi-norm which can be defined as:

$$\|\mathbf{x}\|_0 = \lim_{p \to 0} \sum_i |x_i|^p \tag{3.12}$$

This norm simply counts the number of non-zero coefficients in a vector.

Therefore, finding the optimal solution for the signal $\mathbf{x}$ involves solving the ℓ_0 minimization problem

$$(P_0) \text{ minimize } \|\mathbf{\Psi}\mathbf{x}\|_0, \text{ subject to } \|\mathbf{y} - \mathbf{\Phi}\mathbf{x}\|_2 = 0, \tag{3.13}$$

where $\mathbf{\Psi}$ is the sparsifying transform, $\mathbf{y}$ is the measurement vector, and $\mathbf{\Phi}$ is the measurement matrix. For noisy measurements, the equality $\|\mathbf{y} - \mathbf{\Phi}\mathbf{x}\|_2 = 0$ can not be satisfied, therefore the optimization problem (3.13) is modified to

$$(P_{0,\epsilon}) \text{ minimize } \|\mathbf{\Psi}\mathbf{x}\|_0, \text{ subject to } \|\mathbf{y} - \mathbf{\Phi}\mathbf{x}\|_2 \leq \epsilon, \tag{3.14}$$

where ϵ is related to the signal noise level.

The formulation of Eq. (3.13) and (3.14), where one seeks the signal $\mathbf{x}$ whose transformed coefficients are sparse is called analysis-based model [50]. In an alternative formulation one can also directly seek the sparse coefficients that explain the measurements which can be writen as:

$$(P_0) \text{ minimize } \|\mathbf{z}\|_0, \text{ subject to } \|\mathbf{y} - \mathbf{A}\mathbf{z}\|_2 = 0, \tag{3.15}$$

and

$$(P_0, \epsilon) \text{ minimize } \|\mathbf{z}\|_0, \text{ subject to } \|\mathbf{y} - \mathbf{A}\mathbf{z}\|_2 \leq \epsilon. \tag{3.16}$$

Here $\mathbf{A}$ is the matrix mapping the sparse coefficients $\mathbf{z}$ to the measurement vector $\mathbf{y}$. This formulation is known as the synthesis model.

For orthonormal transforms $\mathbf{\Psi}$ with $\mathbf{A} = \mathbf{\Phi}\mathbf{\Psi}^H$ the synthesis and analysis models are identical. But in general they lead to different solutions [50, 51].

While exact determination of the sparsest solution proves to be an NP-hard problem [52], different techniques have been developed that give a very accurate and sometimes even exact solution of (P_0).

During the last years, many reconstruction algorithms for compressed sensing have been proposed. A main class of sparse recovery algorithms is related to the basis pursuit (BP) or basis pursuit denoising (BPDN) [53]. These methods suggest a convex relaxation of the problems posed in P_0 and $P_{0,\epsilon}$, by replacing the ℓ_0-norm with an ℓ_1-norm. If the isometry constant is small and the signal sparse enough, the ℓ_1-norm minimization provides an exact solution [54].

Another group of algorithms for solving P_0 and $P_{0,\epsilon}$ are greedy algorithms like Matching Pursuit [55]. These methods involve the computation of inner products between the signal and the columns of the matrix $\mathbf{A}$, and possibly deploying some least squares solvers or projections. Similar conditions for exact reconstruction have been derived for these methods [56].

Minimization of non-convex ℓ_p-norms ($0 \leq p < 1$) has been shown to provide a potentially better recovery than ℓ_1 norms [57]. These algorithms are usually based on the iteratively reweighted least squares (IRLS) method [58]. Early work on IRLS methods apply ℓ_p norms with $1 < p < 2$ [59, 60]. Extensions to non-convex optimization frameworks were proposed in [57, 61, 62]. A similar reweighting approach for ℓ_1-norms is proposed in [51].

Iterative shrinkage algorithms are relatively simple methods that could approximate either ℓ_1 or ℓ_0 minimization problems [63–66]. These methods have relatively low computational complexity, which makes them suitable for large scale problems.

In the following, these classes of algorithms will be briefly discussed.

3.2.5.1 ℓ_1-minimization

The Basis Pursuit (BP) algorithm [53] relaxes the ℓ_0 minimization problem in P_0 and $P_{0,\epsilon}$ to an ℓ_1 minimization problem:

$$(P_1) \text{ minimize } \|\mathbf{z}\|_1, \text{ subject to } \|\mathbf{y} - \mathbf{A}\mathbf{z}\|_2 = 0, \tag{3.17}$$

$$(P_{1,\epsilon}) \text{ minimize } \|\mathbf{z}\|_1, \text{ subject to } \|\mathbf{y} - \mathbf{A}\mathbf{z}\|_2 \leq \epsilon, \tag{3.18}$$

Although the ℓ_1 norm is different from the ℓ_0 norm, if the signal is sufficiently sparse and the measurement matrix has small global restricted isometry constants, the ℓ_1 minimization often finds the sparsest solution [33, 67].

Equations (3.17) and (3.18) are convex optimization problems that can be formulated as a linear program and a second order cone program, respectively, and solved by conventional solvers [68]. Although standard solvers can be used for the ℓ_1 minimization problem, solving large-scale problems such as the problems arising in medical imaging is challenging. Since CS was introduced, there has been an increased interest in developing special purpose algorithms for solving of the ℓ_1 minimization problem and there is vast literature on this subject.

The ℓ_1 minimization can be alternatively formulated as an unconstrained problem using the Lagrange form:

$$\operatorname{argmin}_z \|\mathbf{y} - \mathbf{Az}\|_2^2 + \lambda \|\mathbf{z}\|_1 \tag{3.19}$$

and solved using nonlinear conjugate gradients method [69]. Here the regularization parameter λ determines the trade-off between the data consistency and sparsity. Other methods that approximate the ℓ_1 - minimization include projection onto convex sets [70], iterative soft thresholding [58], iteratively reweighted least squares [62], and homotopy [71].

Second-order methods such as interior-point methods [72, 73] offer high accuracy, but need to solve large systems of linear equations to compute the Newton steps, which makes them impractical for large-scale problems. First order methods may be faster, but may require many iterations to achieve high accuracy.

The ℓ_1-minimization approach provides uniform guarantees over all sparse signals and also stability and robustness under measurement noise and approximately sparse signals, but relies on optimization which has relatively high complexity.

3.2.5.2   Greedy Algorithms

Another main group of reconstruction approaches is using greedy algorithms such as the Matching Pursuit (MP) [55]. These algorithms include Orthogonal Matching Pursuit (OMP) [74], Stagewise Orthogonal Matching Pursuit (StOMP) [75], Regularized Orthogonal Matching Pursuit [76] (ROMP), and Compressive Sampling Matching Pursuit (CoSaMP) [77], just to name a few.

Most of these approaches calculate the support of the signal iteratively. With the support Ω of the signal calculated, the signal can be reconstructed from its measurements by a least squares fit. For the synthesis model, the sparse vector $\mathbf{z}$ is computed as $\mathbf{z} = (\mathbf{A}_\Omega)^+\mathbf{y}$, where $\mathbf{A}_\Omega$ denotes the matrix $\mathbf{A}$ restricted to the columns indexed by Ω and $^+$ denotes the pseudoinverse.

Greedy approaches are relatively fast compared with the Basis Pursuit algorithm but most of them deliver smaller recoverable sparsity compared to ℓ_1 minimization and most of them often come without provable uniform guarantees and stability, with the exception of [76, 77].

As an example of a greedy algorithm for sparse recovery the orthogonal matching pursuit (OMP) algorithm [55, 74, 78] is considered. OMP works iteratively, in each iteration selecting the column of $\mathbf{A}$ having the maximal projection onto the residual signal and adding it to the already selected atoms. After a new column vector is selected, the representation coefficients with respect to the vectors chosen so far are found via least-squares optimization.

Formally, given a measurement vector $\mathbf{y}$ and a matrix $\mathbf{A}$ with normalized columns (in the matching pursuit literature such matrix is called dictionary) the OMP algorithm performs the following steps to estimate the sparse vector $\mathbf{z}$.

Start by setting the residual $\mathbf{r}_0 = \mathbf{y}$, the set of selected columns of $\mathbf{A}$ $\Omega_0 = \emptyset$, and the iteration counter $i = 1$

1. Select the index of the next dictionary element by

$$\omega_i = \operatorname*{argmax}_{j=1,\dots d} |\langle \mathbf{r}_{i-1}, \mathbf{a}_j \rangle|$$

2. Augment the matrix of selected vectors and the selected set of indices

$$\mathbf{A}_{\Omega_i} = \begin{bmatrix} \mathbf{A}_{\Omega_{i-1}} & \mathbf{a}_{\omega_i} \end{bmatrix}$$

$$\Omega_i = \Omega_{i-1} \cup \omega_i$$

3. Update the current estimate

$$\mathbf{z}_i = \operatorname*{argmin}_{\mathbf{z}} \|\mathbf{A}_{\Omega_i} \mathbf{z} - \mathbf{y}\|_2^2$$

4. Update the residual

$$\mathbf{y_i} = \mathbf{A}_{\Omega_i} \mathbf{z}_i$$

$$\mathbf{r_i} = \mathbf{y} - \mathbf{y}_i$$

The algorithm can be stopped after a predetermined number of iterations, hence after having selected a fixed number of atoms. Alternatively, the stopping rule can be based on the norm of the residual.

3.2.5.3   Nonconvex CS algorithms

Several other algorithms replace the ℓ_0 norm with an ℓ_p norm

$$\|\mathbf{x}\|_p = \left(\sum_i |x_i|^p \right)^{1/p} \tag{3.20}$$

In the Focal Under-determined System Solver (FOCUSS) [79], Lagrange multipliers are used to convert the problem to an unconstrained optimization problem, and an iterative method is derived based on the idea of iteratively reweighed least-squares that handles the ℓ_p-norm as a weighted ℓ_2-norm. In FOCUSS, usually $1 \leq p \leq 2$ is used. In [57, 61, 62], the case $p < 1$ is considered. Another reweighted procedure is the iteratively reweighted ℓ_1 minimization [51] in which the solution of the ℓ_1 norm minimization is reweighted to approximate ℓ_0 minimization. The minimization of the ℓ_p norm with $p < 1$ is closer to the original ℓ_0 minimization problem. However, the overall problem becomes non-convex giving rise to local minima and the convergence to a global minimum cannot be guaranteed. An alternative approach is to approximate the ℓ_0 norm by smooth functions [80].

3.2.5.4 Iterative Thresholding/Shrinkage

An alternative class of numerical algorithms addressing the sparse reconstruction problem in a computationally efficient way is the class of iterative shrinkage algorithms [58,63,65,66,81,82]. These methods consist of a multiplication by $\mathbf{A}$ and its adjoint and a shrinkage operation on the sparse vector $\mathbf{z}$.

A simple form of iterative shrinkage can be defined by the following iterations:

$$\mathbf{z}_{i+1} = \mathcal{T}_\lambda(\mathbf{z}_i + \mathbf{A}^T(\mathbf{y} - \mathbf{A}\mathbf{z})) \tag{3.21}$$

where the operator $\mathcal{T}$ is the shrinkage or thresholding operator and λ is the threshold. If the thresholding operator is given by

$$\mathcal{T}_\lambda(\mathbf{x})_i = \begin{cases} \text{sign}(x_i)(|x_i| - \lambda), & \text{if } |x_i| \geq \lambda; \\ 0, & \text{if } |x_i| < \lambda; \end{cases} \tag{3.22}$$

Eq. (3.21) refers to iterative soft thresholding (IST) or if $\mathcal{T}$ is the hard thresholding operator

$$\mathcal{T}_\lambda(\mathbf{x})_i = \begin{cases} x_i, & \text{if } |x_i| \geq \lambda; \\ 0, & \text{if } |x_i| < \lambda; \end{cases} \tag{3.23}$$

(3.21) corresponds to iterative hard thresholding (IHT). There are theoretical results that give sufficient conditions for the IST algorithm to converge to the solution of P_1 [58] and for the IHT algorithm to a local minimum of P_0 [81]. There is a large variety of iterative shrinkage algorithms as they are especially appealing for practical applications of CS. A current review on iterative shrinkage methods can be found in [83].

3.3 CS for MRI

MRI is probably the most advanced technology so far with regards to implementing compressed sensing. Shortly after the first theoretical works on CS, MRI was identified as a potential application that could benefit from the new sampling theorem [70]. This idea was later developed by Lustig et al. [69], who considered practical issues of the acquisition and reconstruction in compressed sensing MRI (CS-MRI). In recent years CS MRI has been a very active research area as evidenced by the rapidly increasing number of conference contributions and journal publications. This section will discuss some basic considerations of the application of CS to MRI.

3.3.1   Sparsity of MR images

The reconstruction of a signal from undersampled linear measurements with CS requires the signal to be sparse. Indeed, some images, like MR angiograms, are already sparse in the image domain. This makes MR angiography a favorable candidate for CS. Most MR images, however, are not sparse in the image domain. In this case sparsity has to be created by applying an appropriate sparsifying transform. Two commonly used transforms in CS-MRI are the finite differences transform and the wavelet transform. These are illustrated in Fig.3.3.

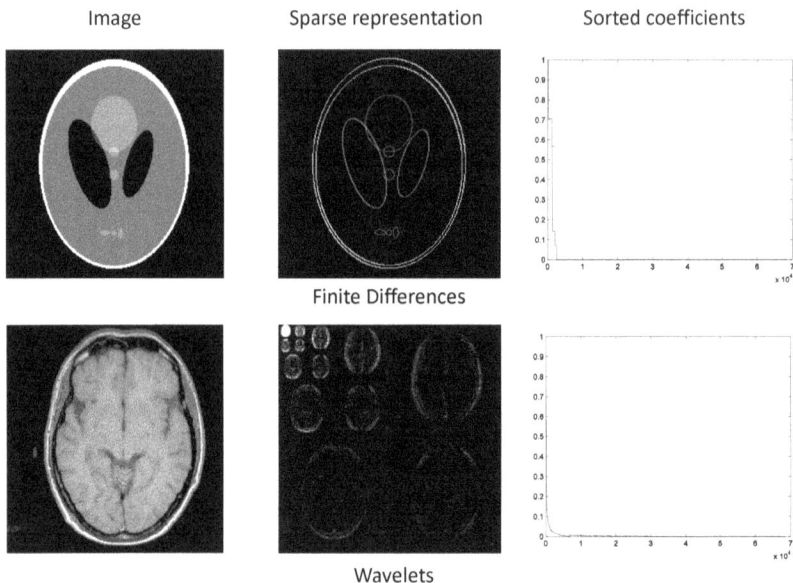

Figure 3.3. Sparsity in different domains. Two sparsifying transforms commonly used in CS MRI are the finite differences and wavelets. Piecewise constant signals such as the Shepp-Logan phantom are extremely sparse in the finite differences transform. In-vivo MRI images are often sparse in the wavelet domain.

Although the finite differences transform truly sparsifies only piecewise constant images like the Shepp-Logan phantom, it is often useful as additional transform in the reconstruction. There are many different wavelet transforms that could be chosen [42], based on properties such as orthogonality and number of vanishing moments or possibly based on some prior knowledge about the class of signals of interest. Sparsity is not limited to single images. In many MRI applications, there are additional signal dimensions in which sparsity can be exploited. This could be a temporal dimension as in dynamic imaging, spectral dimension or a parameter dimension as in MR parameter mapping.

CS allows exact reconstruction only for signals which are exactly sparse. Practical applications deviate from this model in two aspects. First, there is always some measurement noise and since noise is not compressible it prevents the signal from being sparse. Second the signals are often only compressible, which means that instead of zeros they have many small coefficients. In the case of noisy or compressible signals the reconstruction error is proportional to the sparse approximation error, i.e the error obtained when the image is approximated by its S largest coefficients and all the rest is set to zero. Therefore it is instructional to look at the sparse approximation of such signals.

For sparse, but noisy signals setting the small coefficients to zero leads to signal denoising. This is demonstrated on the Shepp-Logan phantom shown in Fig. 3.4.

The sparse approximation of a compressible signal is shown for the example of a brain image in Fig. 3.5. Setting the small wavelet coefficients to zero leads to an approximation error, however up to about a 10% compression this error is hardly perceivable. If too many coefficients are set to zero compression artifacts become visible, which are typically expressed as smoothing and appearance of blocky structures as it can be seen in the image approximated with 5% of the wavelet coefficients in Fig. 3.5.

3.3.2 Sampling and Incoherence in CS-MRI

As discussed in chapter 2, data in MRI are conventionally acquired in the spatial frequency domain, known as k-space. Therefore the measurement matrix Φ is an undersampled Fourier matrix. One could also consider other types of encoding than in the Fourier domain that could possibly improve the incoherence between the sampling and sparsity bases. There are few works suggesting encoding with random matrices [84 86]. Non-Fourier encoding is out of the scope of this work, but it should be kept in mind as an alternative option.

There is a large variety of k-space sampling patterns that could be potentially realized. However, practical considerations set some restrictions such as full sampling in the frequency encoding direction and relatively smooth k-space trajectories due to hardware and physiological constraints.

Because of the restriction to undersampling in the phase encoding direction undersampling in 2D Cartesian imaging can be performed in one dimension only and in 3D Cartesian imaging in two dimensions. Non-Cartesian imaging like radial or spiral allow undersampling in all spatial dimensions and could potentially allow higher undersampling factors. Difficulties using non-Cartesian trajectories include increased computational complexity and higher susceptibility to imperfections in the acquisition such as off-resonance effects, eddy currents and gradient system imperfections.

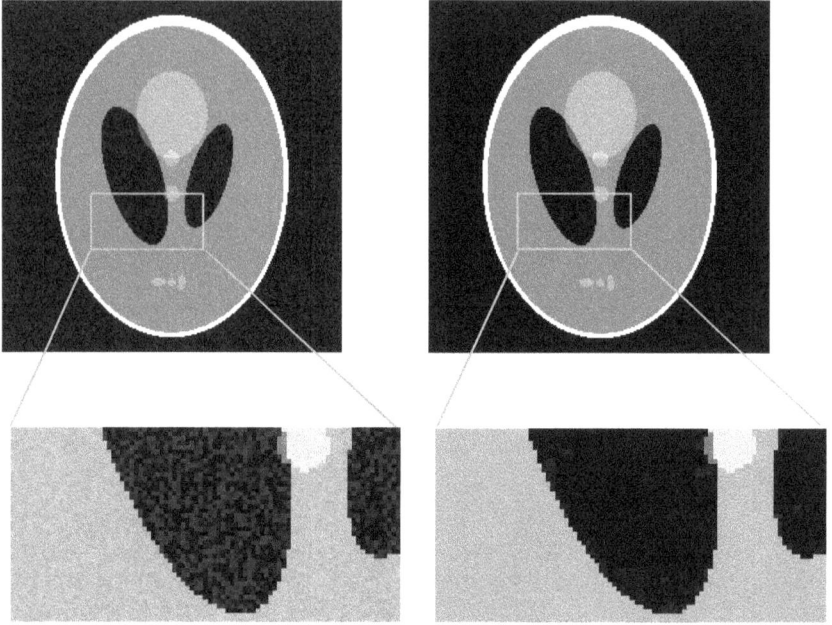

Figure 3.4. Sparse approximation of sparse noisy image. The Shepp-Logan phantom with added Gaussian noise ($\sigma = 0.03$) is approximated with 6% of its coefficients in the wavelet domain (Haar wavelet). The approximated image has reduced noise.

3.3.2.1 Incoherence

From the theoretical point of view random Fourier measurements satisfy the RIP with high probability, which means that if the image is sparse enough it can be reconstructed from a small number of k-space measurements chosen at random. These results are probabilistic, saying that almost any set of k-space measurements will work for almost any signal.

Clearly, among the different realizations of random Fourier sampling some sampling patterns will be better than others. For a fixed sampling pattern (measurement matrix), one can compute the coherence which can be used as the basis for comparison between different sampling patterns. The coherence can also be related to the PSF as suggested in [69]. The PSF for a given measurement matrix $\mathbf{\Phi}$ is defined as:

$$PSF(i,j) = \mathbf{e}_j^H \mathbf{\Phi}^H \mathbf{\Phi} \mathbf{e}_i \tag{3.24}$$

100%   20%   15%

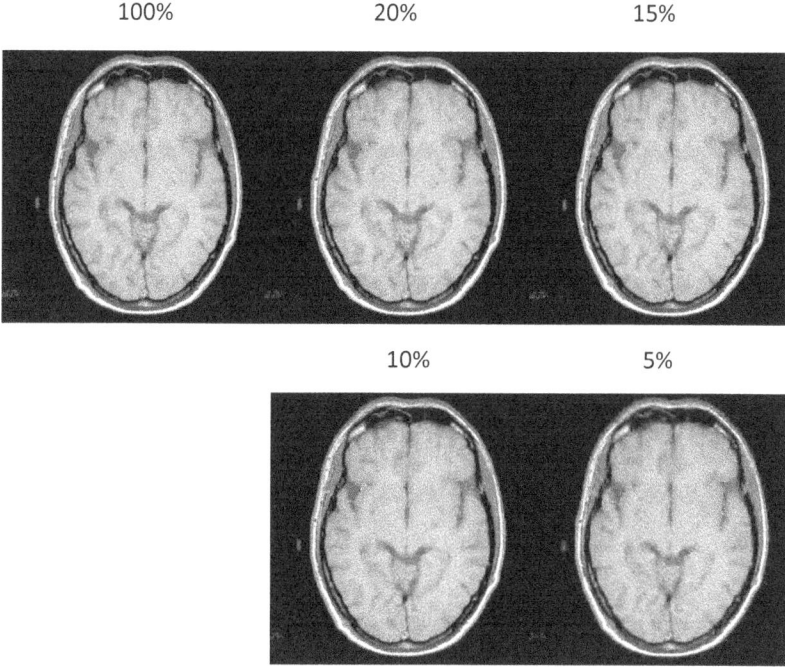

10%   5%

Figure 3.5. Sparse approximation of compressible image. The brain image is approximated by its largest wavelet coefficients (Daubechies 4 wavelet). Signal approximation with 10% of the largest coefficients results in good image quality

where $\mathbf{e}_i$ is the i-th canonical basis vector. For full sampling on a Cartesian grid, the matrix $\boldsymbol{\Phi}$ is orthonormal and all pixels are uncorrelated $PSF(i,j) = \delta(i,j)$. Undersampling causes aliasing, i.e. some of the energy of the main peak leaks to the sidelobes of the PSF. This aliasing pattern shows the correlations between different pixels due to undersampling. The maximum sidelobe-to-peak ratio $SPR(i)$ was introduced by Lustig [69] as a metric to characterize these correlations. It is defined as:

$$SPR(i) = \max_{i \neq j} \frac{PSF(i,j)}{PSF(i,i)} \qquad (3.25)$$

For sparsity in the transform domain $\boldsymbol{\Psi}$, the PSF of the matrix $\mathbf{A} = \boldsymbol{\Phi}\boldsymbol{\Psi}^H$ has to be considered.

which is referred to as transform point spread function $TPSF$ in [69].

$$TPSF(i,j) = \mathbf{e}_j^H \mathbf{A}^H \mathbf{A} \mathbf{e}_i = \mathbf{e}_j^H \boldsymbol{\Psi} \boldsymbol{\Phi}^H \boldsymbol{\Phi} \boldsymbol{\Psi}^H \mathbf{e}_i \qquad (3.26)$$

The maximum SPR is equal to the coherence μ. The coherence is a worst case criterion. It evaluates the maximum correlation between any two coefficients, so if a low coherence sampling is found it will work well for all images. One can imagine a measurement matrix for which two coefficients are highly correlated and all the others are uncorrelated. Such a measurement matrix makes it impossible to distinguish between the two correlated coefficients. However, it is still possible to obtain a perfect reconstruction for all images that do not contain these two coefficients and leads to small reconstruction error for signals which contain these coefficients, but they have small amplitude. On the other hand, for a measurement matrix with the same coherence measure but high correlations between all coefficients it will be impossible to obtain a good reconstruction for any image.

Therefore a metric characterizing the complete aliasing effect pattern might be useful. In this work the mean aliasing energy is intoduced as such metric:

$$MAE(i) = \frac{1}{N} \sum_{i \neq j} \sqrt{\frac{TPSF(i,j)^* TPSF(i,j)}{TPSF(i,i)^* TPSF(i,i)}} \qquad (3.27)$$

that also takes into account the total aliasing due to undersampling.

In the most general case one has to compute the $TPSF$ for each coefficient to obtain the coherence. Although this is much less computationally intensive than verifying the RIP, for typical image sizes it still involves a large number of computations. For example, a relatively small image of 256×256 pixels requires the computation of $256^4 = 4 * 10^9$ coefficients. In the case of sparsity in the image domain, because of the properties of the Fourier matrix the PSF needs to be computed only at a single pixel, which greatly reduces the number of computations. In the case of sparsity in the wavelet transform the SPR and the MAE are constant within each subband, therefore computing the $TPSF$ for one coefficient from each subband is sufficient.

3.3.2.2   Incorporation of prior knowledge

Prior knowledge about the image can be used to design sampling patterns that are appropriate for a given class of images. The maximum incoherence between the canonical basis and the Fourier basis means that if the signal is sparse in the image domain the signal energy is spread in k-space. In this case uniform density random sampling in k-space is appropriate. However, most MR images are not sparse in the image domain, but in some other basis, e.g. wavelets. Usually the significant wavelet components are concentrated around the coarse scales, which are corresponding to the low frequencies. In the Fourier domain this means that the signal energy is usually highest around the k-space origin and decreases toward the edges. This prior knowledge can be used in designing sampling patterns by constructing random sampling patterns according to a probability density function (PDF) with higher density around the k-space origin. In [69], a sampling density according to a power of a distance from the origin was proposed, with density powers of 1 to 6 resulting in greatly improved image quality compared to uniform random sampling.

K-space sampling	SPR wavelets	Aliasing in image space

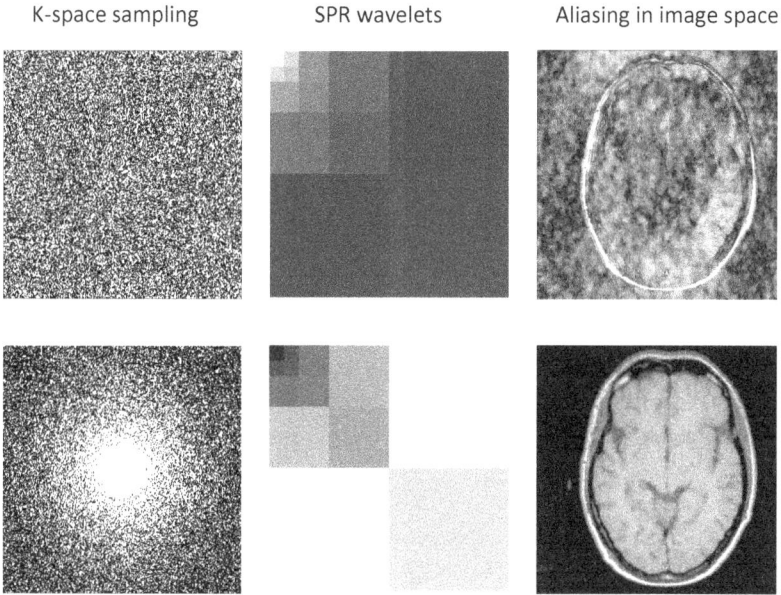

Figure 3.6. Variable density sampling. Random sampling with uniform and with variable sampling density are considered. The distribution of the SPR in the wavelet domain shows that the uniform density sampling pattern results in high correlations between the coarse scale coefficients, while for variable density sampling the high correlations are in the fine scale coefficients. Therefore for an image, in which most of the energy is concentrated in the coarse scale wavelet coefficients, the variable density sampling results in much less artifacts.

Using a variable density sampling pattern does not necessarily improve the incoherence. However it does change the correlations between different coefficients. Fig. 3.6 shows an example of two random sampling patterns, one with uniform density and one with variable density. The $TPSF$ was computed for each wavelet coefficient for the two sampling patterns. The maximum SPR for each wavelet coefficient is shown in Fig. 3.6. The coherence is $\mu = 0.116$ for the uniform density and $\mu = 0.149$ for the variable density sampling. The mean aliasing energy is $MAE = 0.0475$ and $MAE = 0.0498$ for the uniform and the variable density case, respectively. Based on these metrics there is no reason why variable density sampling should be preferred. The reason can better be understood by looking at the distribution of the correlations between the coefficients in the sparsity domain. It can be seen that in the uniform density case the highest correlations are for the coarse scale coefficients, while in the variable density case these are shifted to the fine scale coefficients. Although the coherence for the variable density sampling is higher, since the high coherence is in the fine scale coefficients, it results in smaller aliasing artifacts for an image with low energy in the fine scale coefficients, like the brain image shown in Fig. 3.6. Therefore the variable sampling density is advantageous only for signals corresponding to the assumed distribution. An even more adaptive scheme was proposed in [87] suggesting that the PDF is determined according to the energy distribution of a separately acquired reference scan.

3.3.2.3 How many samples to acquire?

Theoretical bounds on the number of samples that need to be acquired in order to be able to reconstruct any S-sparse signal are derived in [34, 54]. The two main factors influencing the number of required samples are the signal sparsity and the sampling matrix coherence. In MRI the images we are interested in are lying in a very small subspace of the high dimensional space they are occupying. Often additional prior knowledge is used in choosing the sampling pattern as described in the previous section. This implies that the theoretical bounds do not strictly apply in this case, because we are interested in reconstructing a given subset of images, therefore the influence of the coherence is reduced. Empirical results show that one can achieve a good reconstruction if 2 to 5 times the number of sparse coefficients are acquired.

A fundamental lower limit of the number of samples that need to be acquired is the number of sparse coefficients S. Even if the locations of the sparse coefficients are known, one cannot reconstruct the image from less than S samples. Since these locations are in general unknown and have to be recovered by the reconstruction, at least $2S$ measurements need to be performed. Depending on the reconstruction method, the coherence of the sampling pattern, and on the accuracy of the prior knowledge used some more measurements might be needed.

Therefore, the main factor which determines the number of necessary samples is the signal sparsity. Usually MR images are not strictly sparse but rather compressible in some transform domain. The signal sparsity can be determined by the number of coefficients which are sufficient to approximate the image without degrading its diagnostic quality.

3.3.3 State of the art in CS-MRI

Future acceptance of compressed sensing in MRI will depend on whether it proves to be more efficient than other acceleration strategies. Likely, this will only be achieved by combining compressed sensing with existing acceleration strategies and specifically parallel imaging. Therefore, an investigation of the synthesis of compressed sensing and parallel imaging, and in particular how the two associated reconstruction methods may efficiently interact with each other, is of high relevance. The scan acceleration in compressed sensing and parallel imaging relies on completely different principles. In parallel imaging, it is mainly determined by the properties of the coil array, while in compressed sensing, it is the compressibility of the images that plays the key role. In principle, both types of knowledge can be combined in the reconstruction to reduce the required amount of data further. Several works have been presented [88–92] proposing a combined CS-SENSE reconstruction by adding an ℓ_1 regularization term to the iterative SENSE reconstruction. Liang et al. [93] have proposed a two step approach, first performing CS to obtain a set of uniformly undersampled images and as a second step performing SENSE to reconstruct the final image. A combination of CS with autocalibration parallel imaging reconstruction has been proposed in [94, 95].

Besides the reconstruction method, the sampling strategy is another important issue in CS-PI. Uniform subsampling is usually employed in the acquisition in PI, while an irregular subsampling is used in the acquisition in CS. It has been shown that random sampling with more regular distribution of the sampling points like Poisson disk sampling works works well for both PI and CS [94]. There are also several works applying randomized sampling for PI [87], or using ℓ_1 regularization in regularly undersampled parallel imaging [96].

Accelerating the acquisition process is of major interest for various MRI applications. CS is not intrinsically limited to a certain application, however, its performance, i.e. the achievable scan time reduction, strongly depends on the sparsity or compressibility of the acquired images, which can vary considerably between different applications. In this chapter CS has been considered to speed up the acquisition of a single 2 or 3D image. However, some applications provide additional sampling dimensions, for which different sampling strategies and sparsifying transforms may be advantageous. This motivates considering CS separately for each application.

One application of particular interest is contrast enhanced angiography. Angiograms are already very sparse in the image domain and can be sparsified further using a finite difference transform, enabling a substantial acceleration of the measurement or improvement of the spatial and temporal resolution, which is of high relevance especially in time-resolved angiography [97].

Besides angiography, dynamic cardiac imaging is of great interest [98–100]. Dynamic images are highly compressible in the temporal direction and in CS this compressibility is exploited for scan acceleration.

Relaxation parameter mapping is also of interest because of its often long acquisition times. Similarly to the temporal dimension in dynamic imaging, the parameter dimension provides an additional sampling dimension, which can be used for undersampling. Works in this field include [101–104].

Similar methodology can be employed for scan time reduction in diffusion spectrum imaging [105, 106], phase contrast imaging [107, 108] and Fourier velocity encoded MRI [109], among others.

Compressed sensing is also of considerable interest in hyperpolarized MRI. A major difficulty in hyperpolarized imaging is the short acquisition time restricted by T_1, which limits the spatial resolution. Compressed sensing allows improving the spatial resolution without decreasing the coverage. Hyperpolarized 13C MRSI with CS has been presented in [110, 111] hyperpolarized 3He lung MRI has been considered in [112]. CS has also been applied for chemical shift based water-fat separation [113, 114].

Chapter Four

CS WITH GOLDEN RATIO RADIAL SAMPLING

> *Geometry has two great treasures: one is the theorem of Pythagoras, the other, the division of a line into extreme and mean ratio. The first we may compare to a measure of Gold; the second we may name a precious jewel.*
>
> — JOHANNES KEPLER

Low coherence sampling trajectories are favorable in CS. In Cartesian k-space sampling, incoherence can be accomplished by randomly undersampling the data in the phase encoding direction(s). Therefore, the undersampling is limited to one direction in 2D and two directions in 3D sampling, which limits the achievable acceleration factor. Undersampling in all spatial directions can be achieved using non-Cartesian trajectories. One practical non-Cartesian trajectory, which has low coherence, is radial sampling. In radial sampling, data are usually acquired along lines passing through the k-space origin with uniform angular spacing. This chapter considers CS reconstruction using a radial sampling trajectory with non-uniform angular spacing, in which data are acquired according to the golden ratio. The golden ratio radial sampling reduces the symmetry of the *PSF* in radial sampling and furthermore allows great flexibility in dynamic imaging.

4.1   Introduction

In radial MRI (or projection reconstruction (PR)) data are obtained along lines passing through the k-space origin. It was the first trajectory to be used in MRI by Lauterbur in his seminal paper [4]. Recently, radial imaging has gained new interest for applications like angiography [14, 32] and ultra-short echo time imaging [115].

One advantage of radial sampling is that it is relatively robust with respect to undersampling. In radial undersampling the aliasing appears as slight streaking and increased pseudo-noise, whereas in Cartesian undersampling it results in severe ghost artifacts. Extending the radial sampling to 3D is even more advantageous, because the aliasing energy is distributed over the entire imaging volume leading to lower aliasing amplitudes [14]. Radial trajectories are relatively insensitive to motion because of the frequent resampling of the k-space origin. They are also valuable for imaging tissues with short T_2 relaxation times, because they can be performed with no gradient encoding before the data acquisition begins, starting in the k-space center [116].

These properties of radial sampling are used, among other approaches, for accelerated k-space sampling [14]. Undersampled radial trajectories are often used in dynamic applications to achieve high temporal and high spatial resolution, while tolerating some artifacts. In high contrast applications, such as angiography, the streaking is less prominent and even higher acceleration factors can be achieved [117, 118].

The aliasing in undersampled radial imaging can be reduced by applying prior knowledge about the measured signal in the reconstruction. Highly constrained backprojection for time resolved MRI (HYPR) [32] uses prior knowledge of a high resolution image with no temporal information and the assumption of low resolution dynamic information (i.e. the signals in neighboring pixels have very similar temporal evolution). This helps reducing the aliasing in each radially undersampled time frame, allowing to improve the temporal resolution in MR angiography. Compressed sensing [33, 34], on the other hand, applies more abstract prior knowledge about the signal such as sparsity or compressibility and is therefore applicable to a broader class of applications.

As discussed in section 3.3.2.1, CS requires a sampling pattern, resulting in incoherent noise like artifacts. Practical schemes for low coherence data sampling in MRI can be achieved by randomly skipping phase encoding lines as proposed by Lustig et al. [69]. Such a sampling scheme is easy to implement and refers to the major part of MRI scans, namely Cartesian. However, in Cartesian sampling, the aliasing energy is distributed only in the phase encoding directions (one dimension for 2D and two dimensions for 3D sampling), which is restricting the acceleration factor. Non-Cartesian trajectories, on the other hand, can be applied to achieve undersampling in all measured directions. There are many known non-Cartesian k-space trajectories (see section 2.4.2) and possibly others can be designed that could be considered as potential CS sampling trajectories. Undersampled variable density trajectories like radial and variable density spiral are of special interest, because they naturally provide a variable density k-space coverage. This is often desired because most of the signal energy is usually concentrated near the k-space center (see 3.3.2.2). This work focuses on radial sampling as one of the oldest and most well explored sampling trajectories that is inherently well suited for undersampling. In this chapter, a special case of radial sampling is assessed as a candidate for a practical non-Cartesian CS sampling scheme.

The radial sampling pattern considered here is based on a golden ratio concept. Golden ratio sampling results in a more irregular sampling pattern which can be favorable in CS. It also allows greater freedom in the choice of the time frame in dynamic imaging. With golden ratio sampling the frame length can be adapted to the signal kinetics and could also be determined retrospectively [119]. As an example, the application of compressed sensing for 2D dynamic cardiac imaging and 3D imaging of the hand will be considered.

4.2 Golden ratio radial sampling

A uniformly undersampled radial trajectory achieves undersampling in all measured dimensions. The uniform radial sampling results in a point spread function with oscillatory behavior and peak aliasing amplitude occuring at concentric rings, with radii determined by the maximum distance between two points in the radial k-space trajectory. However, the aliasing amplitude is small, which makes radial sampling a good candidate for a practical CS trajectory. Randomizing the angles at which radial profiles are acquired can be used to obtain a more irregular sampling scheme, and to reduce the symmetries of the uniform radial *PSF*. However, a purely random distribution of the radial profiles tends to build clusters of closely spaced profiles and large gaps between samples, which could increase the aliasing energy of the sampling pattern. In this work, an irregular radial sampling pattern with nearly uniform angular distribution of the radial profiles is considered, which is based on the golden ratio concept.

4.2.1 The golden ratio

The golden ratio can be defined by partitioning a line segment, such that the ratio of the longer to the shorter partition is equal to the ratio of the initial segment to the longer partition:

$$\frac{a}{b} = \frac{a+b}{a} = \varphi \tag{4.1}$$

From equation (4.1) follows that the golden ratio φ can be determined as the positive root of the quadratic equation

$$\varphi^2 - \varphi - 1 = 0, \text{which is} \tag{4.2}$$
$$\varphi = \frac{1+\sqrt{5}}{2}. \tag{4.3}$$

The golden ratio can be used to determine the locations of a series of points on a line segment as shown in Fig. 4.1. The location of the n-th point on the segment is determined as the modulo of $n\varphi$. The pattern thus obtained has the property that at arbitrarily chosen time intervals the sampling points are distributed almost uniformly on the line segment. The golden ratio often occurs in nature as in growing patterns of flowers, shells, and galaxies, and is referred to symmetry of growth, because it allows adding a new element to an already existing arrangement, while preserving the symmetry [120]. Fig. 4.1 (a) illustrates this property by showing the distribution of different number successively selected of points on a line segment, obtained according to the golden ratio. Compared with uniform density random distribution Fig. 4.1 (b) the golden ratio results in more uniform pattern.

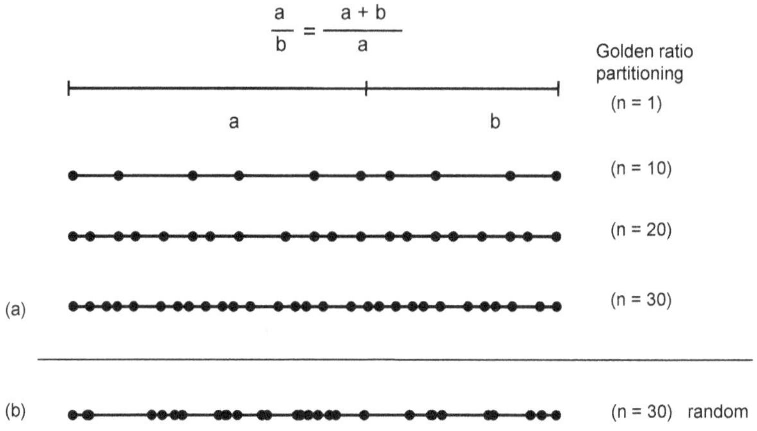

Figure 4.1. Dynamic symmetry of golden ratio sampling. Partitioning according to the golden ratio is shown for a line segment in (a). A new point is always placed on one of the largest segments, such that a nearly uniform distribution is attained at all times. A set of randomly chosen points according to a uniform distribution tends to build clusters and larger gaps, as shown in (b).

4.2.2   2D Golden ratio sampling

A 2D radial trajectory based on the golden ratio was proposed in [119] as an optimal radial view order in dynamic imaging. Data in successively measured radial profiles are acquired at a constant incremental angle based on the golden ratio. The golden angle is determined as

$180°/\varphi \approx 111.246°$. This sampling attains a nearly uniform distribution of the radial profiles in 2D k-space for an arbitrary set of successively acquired profiles. Applied to dynamic imaging, this enables variable frame lengths, which could be determined and selected after the data are measured, as well as arbitrary positions of the time frames.

The distribution of radial profiles in golden ratio sampling is not perfectly uniform, which reduces some of the symmetries of uniformly undersampled radial sampling. This can be seen in Fig. 4.2, which shows the PSF for uniformly undersampled radial sampling and golden ratio sampling with the same number of profiles. For the example shown Fig. 4.2 the mean aliasing energy for the golden ratio sampling is $MAE_{gr} = 3.446 \times 10^{-5}$ and for the uniform radial sampling $MAE_{ur} = 3.451 \times 10^{-5}$. The maximum sidelobe to peak ratio is $SPR_{gr} = 0.030$ and $SPR_{ur} = 0.0345$ for the golden ratio and the uniform radial sampling, respectively. The uniform radial sampling provides lower coherence compared to the golden ratio sampling within a circular FOV, which corresponds for full sampling. However, for a larger FOV (i.e. in case of undersampling), the mean aliasing energy and the maximum sidelobe to peak ratio are lower for the golden ratio sampling. The angular distances between neighboring profiles in golden ratio sampling are concentrated around 3 different angles (or 2 if the number of profiles equals a Fibonacci number), which similarly to the uniform radial sampling results in oscillatory behavior of the PSF, but the aliasing amplitude is decreased.

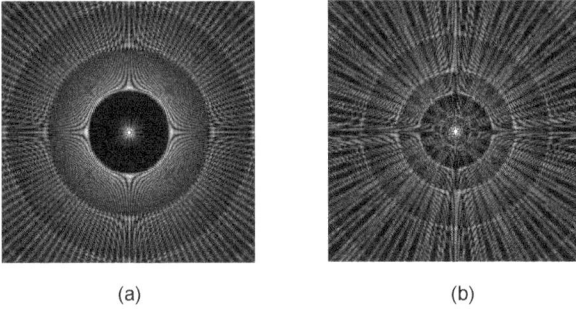

(a)   (b)

Figure 4.2. Undersampling of radial trajectories. The PSF is shown for **(a)** uniformly undersampled radial sampling and **(b)** golden ratio sampling with the same number of radial profiles. The aliasing pattern of the golden ratio radial trajectory is less structured and the aliasing energy is more uniformly distributed over the FOV. The images are enhanced by a factor of 20 for better visualization.

4.2.3 3D Golden ratio sampling

Distributing the radial profiles in three dimensions could potentially allow for higher acceleration factors. A 3D radial sequence that aims for a quasi-isotropic distribution of radial profiles in 3D k-space over the total duration of a scan as well as over an arbitrary time window extracted from scan for dynamic imaging can be achieved by using the golden ratio in two dimensions.

An extension of the golden ratio to multiple dimensions, derived from the extended Fibonacci series, was presented in [121]. The two dimensional golden ratio is determined by two coefficients $\alpha = 0.4656$ and $\beta = 0.6823$, which can be used to distribute a sequence of points on a plane using the coordinates $\mathrm{mod}(n\alpha)$ and $\mathrm{mod}(n\beta)$.

The 3D radial trajectory based on the golden ratio is determined by distributing the tips of the radial profiles on the spherical surface according to the two dimensional golden ratio. This can be achieved by using the increments $\Delta k_z = 2\alpha$ and $\Delta\varphi = 2\pi\beta$ for successively measured profiles, where Δk_z is the increment of k_z and $\Delta\varphi$ is the increment along the polar angle of the projection in the k_x-k_y plane [122]. The 3D golden ratio radial sampling is illustrated in Fig. 4.3. A similar trajectory, for which the profile tips are distributed on a half sphere, is presented in [123].

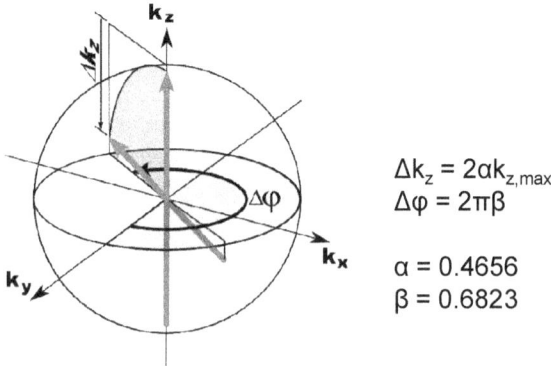

$$\Delta k_z = 2\alpha k_{z,max}$$
$$\Delta\varphi = 2\pi\beta$$

$$\alpha = 0.4656$$
$$\beta = 0.6823$$

Figure 4.3. 3D golden angle sampling. Successive radial profiles are acquired twith increments Δk_z and $\Delta\varphi$, determined by the 2D golden ratio coefficients α and β.

4.3 Reconstruction

As described in section 3.2.5 the CS reconstruction problem can be formulated as an ℓ_1-norm regularized least squares problem:

$$\operatorname*{argmin}_{\mathbf{x}} \|\mathbf{y} - \mathbf{\Phi}\mathbf{x}\|_2^2 + \lambda \|\mathbf{\Psi}\mathbf{x}\|_1, \tag{4.4}$$

where $\mathbf{y}$ is the vector of the measured data, $\mathbf{x}$ is the unknown image, $\mathbf{\Phi}$ is the sampling matrix and $\mathbf{\Psi}$ is the sparsifying transform.

The sampling matrix is the operator, which maps the image $\mathbf{x}$ to the acquired k-space. One can think of the radial MR acquisition as a system, evaluating the radial Fourier transform of an object and the task of the reconstruction is to invert this transform. Using a matrix notation, the forward transform is given by:

$$\mathbf{y} = \mathbf{F}_r\mathbf{x}, \tag{4.5}$$

where $\mathbf{F}_r$ is the radial Fourier transform. The radial Fourier transform can be directly computed as a discrete Fourier transform on the radial grid. For any practical application this approach is too computationally intensive, therefore an approximation using the FFT is used instead. The forward transform is computed by applying an FFT of the image $\mathbf{x}$ and then interpolating the k-space data from the Cartesian to the radial grid using a convolution kernel as described in section 2.4.3. The effects of the convolution with the gridding kernel are compensated in a deapodization step before the FFT. This procedure is sometimes referred to as inverse gridding (the gridding reconstruction is described in section 2.4.3).

If sufficient data are collected and the matrix $\mathbf{F}_r$ is invertible, the image reconstruction from radial data can be obtained as:

$$\mathbf{x} = \mathbf{F}_r^+\mathbf{y} = \left(\mathbf{F}_r^H\mathbf{F}_r\right)^{-1}\mathbf{F}_r^H\mathbf{y}, \tag{4.6}$$

where $\mathbf{F}_r^H$ is the Hermitian radial Fourier transform, consisting of convolution interpolation from the radial to the Cartesian grid, inverse FFT and deapodization. In the gridding reconstruction described in section 2.4.3, the explicit inversion of the matrix $\left(\mathbf{F}_r^H\mathbf{F}_r\right)$ is avoided by applying a preconditioner derived from geometrical reasoning (the density compensation function), which makes the forward transform approximately orthonormal. The reconstruction problem can also be solved iteratively, without using the density compensation function.

In 2D uniform radial sampling, usually $\frac{\pi}{2}N$ radial projections with N samples each are sufficient to assure adequate reconstruction of an $N \times N$ image using conventional reconstruction. This can be related to the Nyquist criterion, applied for the maximum distance between two samples in the radial k-space trajectory. If less samples are acquired, this problem becomes ill conditioned and some additional information is needed to obtain a proper solution.

In this work, compressed sensing is applied for the reconstruction of undersampled radial data, exploiting the signal sparsity to constrain the solution, and the reconstruction problem is formulated as:

$$\text{argmin}_{\mathbf{x}} ||\mathbf{y} - \mathbf{F}_r\mathbf{x}||_2^2 + \lambda ||\mathbf{\Psi x}||_1. \tag{4.7}$$

For data acquired with multiple receive coils, Eq. 4.7 is extended to:

$$\text{argmin}_{\mathbf{x}} \sum_i ||\mathbf{y}_i - \mathbf{F}_r\mathbf{C}_i\mathbf{x}||_2^2 + \lambda ||\mathbf{\Psi x}||_1, \tag{4.8}$$

where $\mathbf{C}_i$ denotes the receive sensitivity of the i-th coil element and $\mathbf{y}_i$ denotes the acquired data from that element. The problems in Eqs. (4.7) and (4.8) can be solved using nonlinear conjugate gradients algorithm as described in [69].

In radial sampling, deviations between the ideal and actual trajectory due to system imperfections (e.g. eddy currents) lead to serious image artifacts, as the signals from different radial profiles do not add coherently at the k-space center. Therefore, the data need to be corrected for k-space misalignments prior to the reconstruction. Misplacements of the trajectory along the readout direction lead to a linear phase in image space. This could be estimated from radial profiles acquired in opposite or approximately opposite directions [124].

4.4   2D golden ratio dynamic cardiac imaging

4.4.1   Experiments

Dynamic cardiac data of a healthy volunteer were acquired with 2D golden ratio radial sampling using a Steady State Free Precession (SSFP) sequence (TR = 2.59 ms, FOV = 350×350 mm^2, 192×192 matrix, 8 mm slice thickness, flip angle 60°, 5 element cardiac receive coil) on a 1.5T clinical scanner. Data were collected during free breathing for 10 s.

To determine the necessary temporal resolution, a series of images with varying temporal resolution were reconstructed from the data using conventional gridding reconstruction as illustrated in Fig. 4.4. The selected time frame contained 32, 55, 89, 144, and 233 projections, resulting in a temporal resolutions of 83, 142, 230, 373, and 602 ms, respectively. To obtain images at different time points the frame can be shifted in steps of one or more TR.

Based on the selected temporal resolution, the dynamic dataset was divided in time frames containing 32 radial profiles each, which corresponds to temporal resolution of 83 ms. The images for each frame were reconstructed with gridding reconstruction and with CS. In the CS reconstruction, the finite differences transform was applied as a sparsifying transform in the image domain. Sparsity in the temporal domain was introduced using temporal differences operator, which computes a difference between the image in the current time frame and an image from a larger time frame centered at the same position (see Fig. 4.4 (b)). The reconstruction

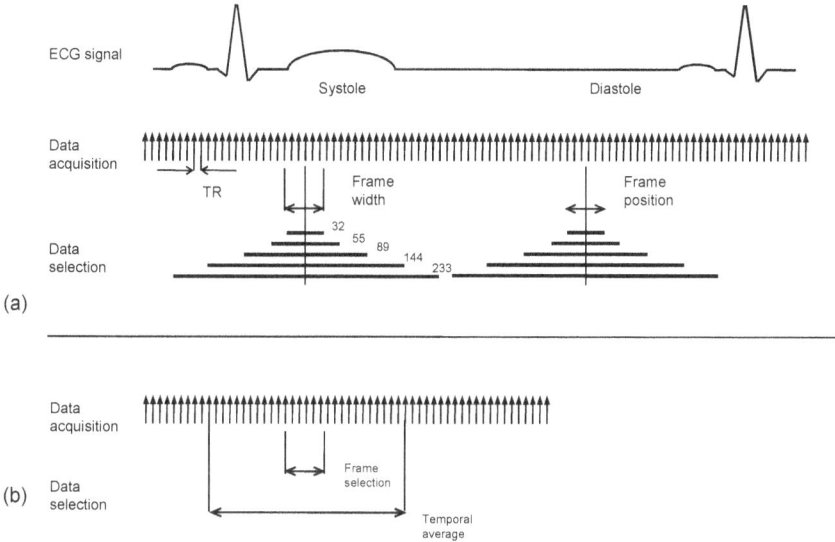

Figure 4.4. Temporal resolution in golden ratio sampling. **(a)** The temporal resolution in golden ratio sampling can be adjusted retrospectively by varying the width of the time frame used in the reconstruction. The frame position and frame width can be varied in steps of one or more TR. **(b)** The image in the current time frame can be sparsified by subtracting a temporal average image obtained from a larger time centered at the same position.

was performed by solving the minimization problem:

$$\operatorname*{argmin}_{\mathbf{x}} \sum_i ||\mathbf{y}_i - \mathbf{F}_r\mathbf{C}_i\mathbf{x}||_2^2 + \lambda_1||\mathbf{D}\mathbf{x}||_1 + \lambda_2||\mathbf{x} - \mathbf{x}_0||_1, \qquad (4.9)$$

where $\mathbf{D}$ is a finite differences transform and $\mathbf{x}_0$ is a temporal average image, obtained from a larger time frame around the current time frame.

An estimation for the relative coil sensitivities was obtained similarly to the method described in [125] by reconstructing images using the complete dynamic dataset for each coil element and dividing each image by the combined sum of squares image. Alternatively, coil sensitivity estimates can be obtained from the central part of k-space, or from a separate reference scan.

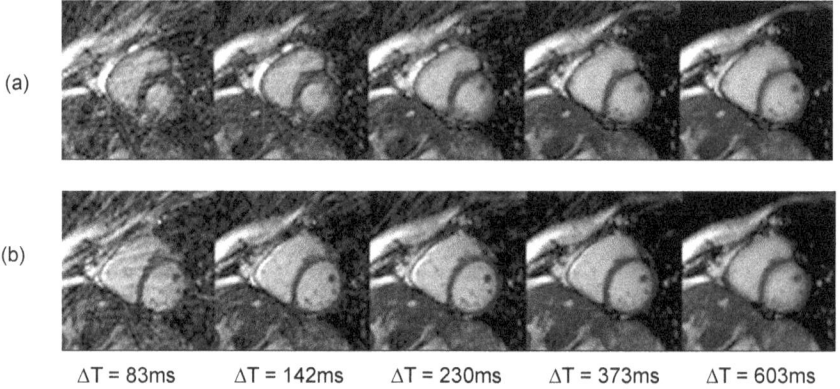

ΔT = 83ms ΔT = 142ms ΔT = 230ms ΔT = 373ms ΔT = 603ms

Figure 4.5. Temporal resolution and aliasing in golden ratio sampling. **(a)** a selected systolic and **(b)** diastolic cardiac phase (short axis view) is shown, reconstructed from frames with different lengths ΔT. Using a short frame length allows more accurate depiction of the actual cardiac phase at the cost of streaking artifacts.

4.4.2 Results

Figure 4.5 shows the images for the systolic (a) and the diastolic (b) phase with different temporal resolutions reconstructed with gridding reconstruction and combined using the estimated coil sensitivities [17]. At high temporal resolution, the images accurately depict the actual cardiac phase. However, they are corrupted by streaking artifacts due to undersampling. Increasing the frame length results in reduced aliasing, but the reconstructed images exhibit temporal blurring over many cardiac phases. Thus, the image content can significantly deviate from the cardiac phase, at which the frame is centered. This effect is stronger in the systolic phase due to the faster cardiac motion. Therefore, for accurate imaging of the cardiac motion, it is necessary to use a short frame length to freeze motion sufficiently. For the given dataset a temporal resolution of 83 ms was chosen.

Images from the dynamic dataset, reconstructed at a temporal resolution of 83 ms, for different cardiac phases are shown in Fig. 4.6. Figures 4.6 (a) and (b) show the images obtained with gridding reconstruction and with CS reconstruction, respectively. The images, reconstructed with CS show significant reduction of the streaking artifacts, improving the image quality.

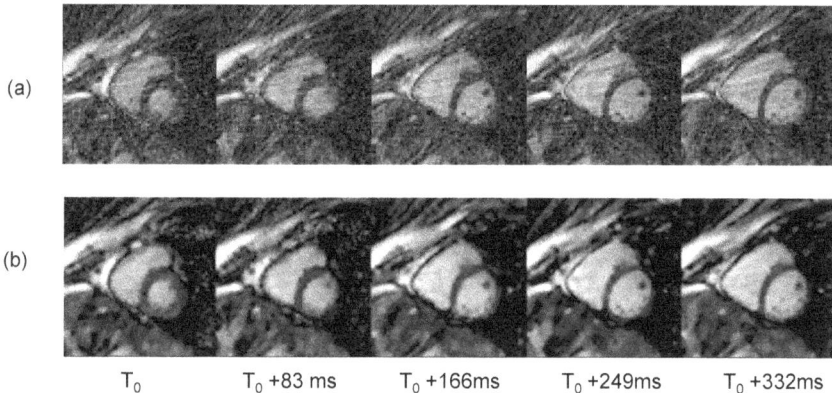

(a)

(b)

T_0 T_0 +83 ms T_0 +166ms T_0 +249ms T_0 +332ms

Figure 4.6. Reconstruction of dynamic cardiac data at high temporal resolution. Images of the dynamic dataset reconstructed at temporal resolution of $\Delta T = 83$ ms are shown obtained with **(a)** gridding reconstruction **(b)** compressed sensing. The CS reconstruction shows improved image quality.

4.5   3D golden ratio sampling

4.5.1   Experiments

To illustrate the capability to resolve motion in volumetric data, 3D radial data with golden ratio sampling were acquired during continuous hand motion using the following parameters: TE $= 0.87$ ms, TR $= 4.0$ ms, flip angle $10°$, FOV $256 \times 256 \times 256$ mm^3, matrix $128 \times 128 \times 128$. Data were acquired on a 1.5T clinical scanner and partitioned in frames with 1365 profiles each, corresponding to a temporal resolution of $\Delta T = 5.4$ s. Images from each time frame were obtained with conventional gridding reconstruction and with CS using finite differences and wavelets (Daubechies 4) as a sparsifying transform.

Furthermore, to study the ability of undersampling in 3D radial measurements, a full 3D dataset of a static hand was acquired with golden ratio sampling. The dataset was retrospectively undersampled by taking a subset of successively measured radial profiles. The images were reconstructed with gridding reconstruction and with CS for several different undersampling factors.

For imaging of tissues with short T2 components the data acquisition has to be performed as early as possible after excitation. Ultrashort echo time (UTE) sequences [126,127] allow echo times substantially shorter than 1 ms. With these sequences short T_2 tissues like tendons and ligaments can be visualized. To avoid slice selection problems for ultrashort echo time imaging 3D radial sequences are employed [115]. To highlight the fast relaxing components, data at two different echo times are acquired (one dataset is acquired at an ultrashort echo time and the other at a longer echo time at which the signal from the short T2 tissues has decayed) and as a post processing step a difference image is computed. To avoid errors due to chemical shift, the second echo time is selected such that water and fat spins are in-phase.

The 3D golden ratio radial sampling was applied for the acquisition of UTE data of a hand, using the following parameters: $TE_1 = 74$ μs , $TE_2 = 4.5$ ms (corresponding to water-fat in-phase at 1.5 T), TR = 7.1 ms, FOV = $256 \times 256 \times 256$ mm^3, matrix $128 \times 128 \times 128$ $\alpha = 10°$, single channel head coil. Images with different undersampling factors were reconstructed with gridding reconstruction and with CS, applying finite differences (TV) and wavelets (Daubechies 4) as sparsifying transforms.

4.5.2   Results

A selected slice from the 3D images obtained from the reconstruction of the dynamic dataset is shown for several time frames in Fig. 4.7. Each image is reconstructed from a set of sequentially acquired profiles, with a reduction factor of 19. The images, obtained with CS reconstruction show significantly improved image quality compared to the gridding reconstruction. The streaking artifacts are suppressed, and structures in the images are preserved. A 3D surface rendered image of the hand, obtained from the CS reconstructed dataset, is shown for better visualization of the hand motion.

The results of the undersampling experiments of the static hand image are shown in Fig. 4.8. Figure 4.8 shows images reconstructed from undersampled data using gridding and CS as well as fully sampled low resolution images from the same amount of k-space data. In the images reconstructed with CS, streaking artifacts that are prominent in the gridding reconstruction images are significantly suppressed. Up to an undersampling factor of approximately 20, image resolution is relatively well preserved. With increasing data reduction factors the local contrast is decreased, which might result in a loss of low contrast features.

Results from the UTE undersampling experiments are shown in Fig. 4.9. Similarly to the results shown in Fig. 4.8, the CS reconstruction shows decreased streaking for all reduction factors, improving the visualization of the tendons.

4.6   Discussion

The feasibility of the golden ratio radial sampling as a practical CS trajectory was investigated in this chapter. The golden ratio radial trajectory enables irregular variable density sampling with undersampling in all measurement dimensions. Compared with the uniformly undersampled radial trajectory, golden ratio results in more noise-like artifacts, while not significantly increasing the aliasing energy. These features of the golden ratio sampling make it an appropriate sampling pattern for CS, allowing for high undersampling ratios.

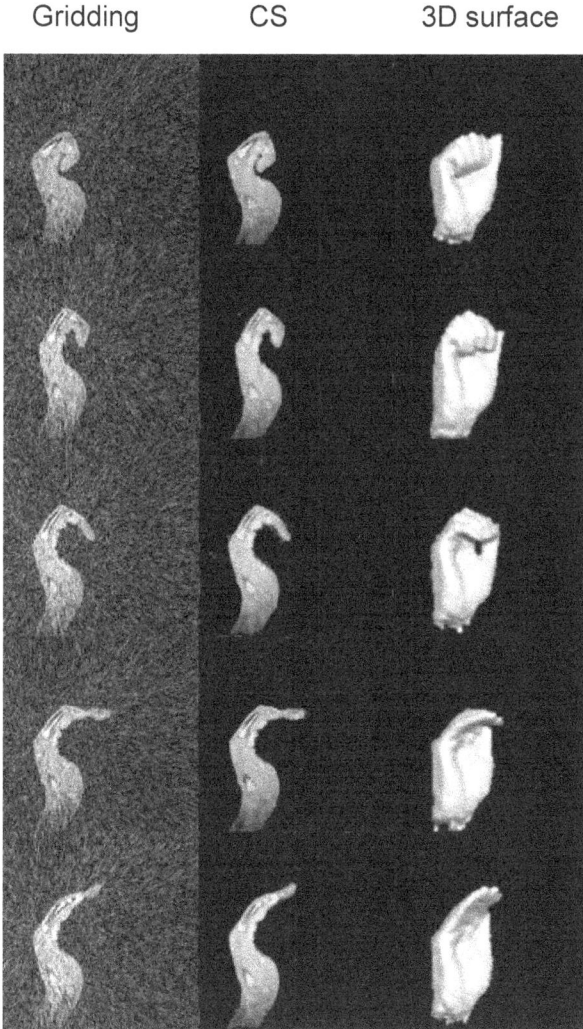

Figure 4.7. 3D golden ratio sampling dynamic hand imaging. The results of conventional gridding reconstruction and compressed sensing are shown for selected time frames using an undersampling factor of 19. Additionally, 3D surface rendered representations of the 3D CS reconstructed images are shown for better visualization of the hand motion. The CS reconstruction results in suppressed streaking and improved image quality.

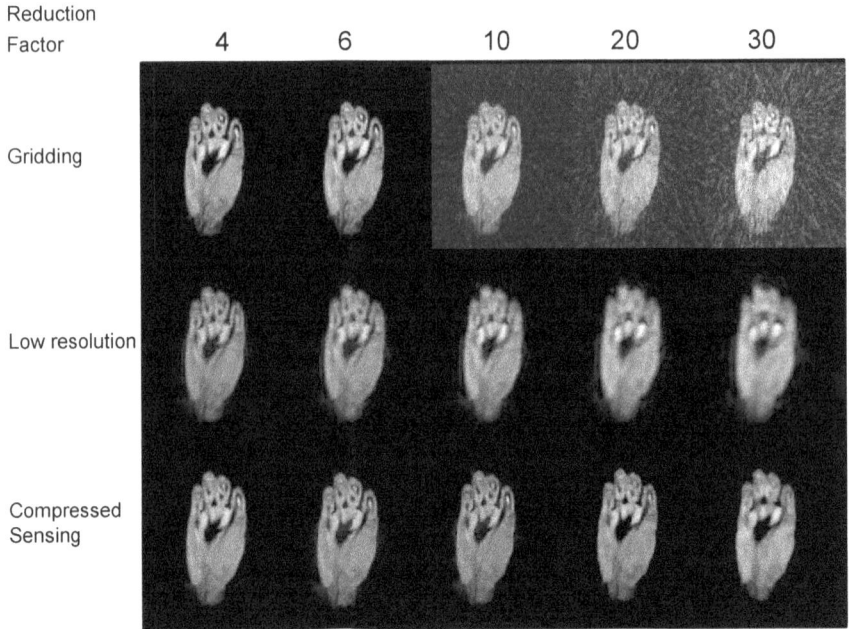

Figure 4.8. 3D golden ratio undersampling. A slice, selected from the 3D images reconstructed from reduced k-space data is shown for different reduction factors. The cutting plane consists of fingers and the major palm muscle structures. CS results in reduced aliasing and high image quality for modest reduction factors. At very high accelerations there is decrease in local contrast and resolution.

Moreover, golden ratio sampling allows relatively uniform coverage of k-space for arbitrarily positioned time frames with arbitrary frame length. This is a desirable property in dynamic imaging, allowing retrospective adjustment of the frame length and position according to the necessary temporal resolution of a dynamic scan. CS using golden ratio sampling was demonstrated in 2D and 3D dynamic imaging experiments with high undersampling factors. The improvement in image quality facilitates high temporal resolution in dynamic imaging, which is otherwise compromised by streaking artifacts.

In the 2D dynamic cardiac imaging experiments temporal resolution of 83 ms was achieved maintaining a good image quality. The ability of 3D radial sampling to support undersampling in all three spatial dimensions furthermore leads to a better aliasing distribution and and thus to higher achievable undersampling ratios. Dynamic imaging of the hand was obtained with a temporal resolution of 5.4 s.

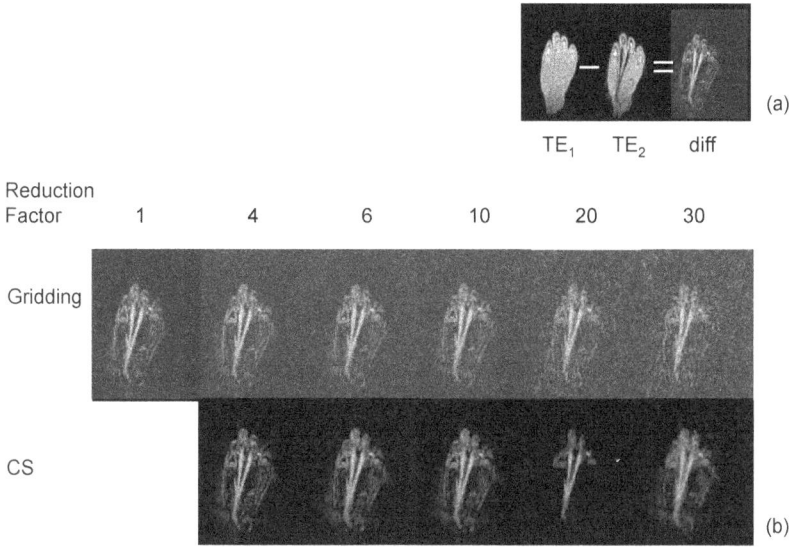

Figure 4.9. UTE imaging with 3D golden ratio sampling. Images of the tendons are obtained with UTE for several different reduction factors as a difference between images at two echo times (see text). The images, obtained using gridding and CS are shown for each reduction factor.

Although the presented results are encouraging, there are several issues that might be limiting for the practical application. CS in 3D radial sampling is challenging because of the high memory requirements and long reconstruction times. The reconstruction times for the examples considered in this chapter were about 30 s for a single frame in 2D imaging and 1 hour for a single 3D image. The 2D experiments were performed with multi-coil acquisition and combined parallel imaging - CS reconstruction. In 3D radial sampling a combination with parallel imaging is currently infeasible because of the long reconstruction times. Fast reconstruction algorithms and dedicated hardware are therefore necessary to address this problem.

Another issue in radial sampling is that due to system imperfections the actual measurements can deviate from the desired trajectory. This is especially apparent in the k-space center, which is resampled in each radial profile. This problem is partly addressed by applying a phase correction before the image reconstruction to correct for profile misalignments. However, more accurate knowledge of the trajectory can further improve the reconstruction.

CHAPTER FIVE

CS PARAMETER MAPPING

The sciences do not try to explain, they hardly even try to interpret, they mainly make models. By a model is meant a mathematical construct which, with the addition of certain verbal interpretations,describes observed phenomena. The justification of such a mathematical construct is solely and precisely that it is expected to work.

— JOHN VON NEUMANN

Signal sparsity is a crucial factor in CS, which determines the achievable undersampling factor. MR images are usually not sparse in the image domain, so a sparsifying transform has to be applied in the CS reconstruction. Prior knowledge about the images is available in many MR applications, which can be exploited to find a sparsifying transform that is tailored to the specific application. In this work it is shown that such prior knowledge permits designing a model-based sparsifying transform that exploits the signal compressibility in MR parameter mapping. The model based transform is applied in compressed sensing reconstruction to accelerate the measurements in MR parameter mapping. The method is presented and evaluated in simulations and in-vivo measurements, exemplified for T_1 and T_2 mapping experiments in the brain. Accurate T_1 and T_2 maps are obtained from highly reduced data. This model-based reconstruction can potentially also be applied to other MR parameter mapping applications like diffusion and perfusion imaging.

Based upon: M. Doneva, C. Stehning, J. Sénégas, P. Börnert, H. Eggers and A. Mertins, "Compressed Sensing Reconstruction for MR parameter mapping", *Magn Reson Med, published online.*

5.1   Introduction

D ifferent tissues in the human body can be distinguished in MRI by their intrinsic MR parameters, such as proton density, longitudinal (T_1) and transversal (T_2) relaxation times [128]. By altering the scanning parameters, such as repetition time (TR), echo time (TE) and flip angle (α), the combined effect of the MR parameters on the image can be changed to obtain different image contrasts. However, such an approach is purely qualitative. Direct quantification of the local MR parameters often provides more accurate and reproducible diagnostic information [129]. MR parameter mapping is, therefore, of interest in a wide range of clinical applications including oncology, neurology and cardiology [129–131].

A major concern in MR parameter mapping is the often long scan time. This has led to an estimation of T_1 and T_2 relaxation times from three or even only two data points, which entails poor accuracy and does not give any indication of multi-compartmental signal behavior. Higher numbers of measurements are necessary to cover a large dynamic range of tissue parameters relevant in clinical applications [132, 133] and also to improve the accuracy of the fit and the SNR.

This chapter presents a technique for reducing the acquisition time in multi-point MR parameter mapping experiments, which is inspired by the theory of compressed sensing. By exploiting the inherent compressibility of MR images, CS allows data reduction without significantly compromising image quality [69]. The compressed sensing recovery algorithms are generic in the sense that they do not assume any other structure in the signal besides its sparsity in some transform domain. The underlying sparsifying transforms are often chosen with very little assumptions about the MR signal. Finite differences and wavelet transforms assume, for instance, that most medical images are piecewise smooth or have sparse wavelet representations. Although these transforms are useful for many signals, they generally allow only modest signal compression, and therefore limited data reduction when used in CS.

The reconstruction could be better tailored to the specific problem if data-specific transforms were used. For example, in dynamic imaging, data are acquired in k–t space to obtain a series of images of a dynamic process. Such data are often highly compressible in the temporal dimension. Sparsity along the temporal dimension is promoted by subtracting a composite image [134] or applying a Fourier transform [98] in case of periodic motion. Related works have been presented for the application in cardiac and functional brain imaging [98, 99, 135].

In this work, the prior knowledge of the data model in MR parameter mapping is used to design a sparsifying transform, which is applied to sparsify the data in CS image reconstruction. Two different model-based sparsifying transforms are presented. The first transform is an orthonormal basis, constructed using principal component analysis (PCA) [136]. The second is an overcomplete dictionary, learned from the data model using a method for overcomplete dictionary design called K-SVD [137]. The proposed method is applicable for MR parameter mapping measurements of T_1 or T_2 relaxation times and diffusion coefficients, among others.

The method is not restricted to exponential models and could potentially be applied to more complex processes like contrast agent uptake and perfusion, in which the signal may also be described by a model.

5.2   Signal model and training data

In the following, the framework of a generalized MR parameter mapping problem will be considered. Given an underlying model $f(p; \boldsymbol{\theta})$, a spatially resolved estimation of the parameters of interest $\boldsymbol{\theta}$ requires the acquisition of several images at different values of the encoding parameter p. A typical data acquisition scheme with Cartesian sampling is shown in Fig. 5.1. This measurement space will be referred to as k–p space. Scan time reduction can be achieved by undersampling in the phase-encoding (k_y) and parameter-encoding (p) dimensions.

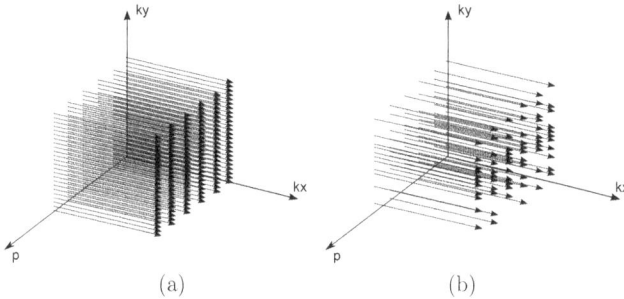

Figure 5.1. Data acquisition in Cartesian k–p space. **(a)** Conventional sampling where a full Cartesian dataset is acquired for each acquisition parameter value p. **(b)** Incoherent sampling for compressed sensing, achieved by variable density random undersampling of phase encodes with higher density near the k–space origin. In this way the data acquisition time can be reduced.

Knowledge of the data model allows generating a set of signal prototypes by evaluating the model for a discrete set of parameters. This set of prototype signals characterizes the data dependencies within the model and could be used as a training set to design a model-adapted sparsifying transform. Generating the training set requires only knowledge of the model and the expected range of the parameters, but no previously measured data are necessary.

Fig. 5.2 illustrates how the training data set is formed. Given a set of sampling locations along the encoding parameter p and a sample value of the parameters $\boldsymbol{\theta}$ a signal prototype $\mathbf{s}$ can be generated by evaluating the function values $f(p; \boldsymbol{\theta})$ at the given parameter values. Performing such an evaluation for different parameter values $\boldsymbol{\theta}$ provides a set of prototypes (examples) $\mathbf{s}_j(i) = f(p_i, \boldsymbol{\theta_j})$, which can be grouped in the matrix $\mathbf{S}$. Each column of the matrix $\mathbf{S}$ forms a discrete signal prototype. Training data $\mathbf{S}$ can be generated based on a uniformly distributed set of parameter values in the expected range. For instance, the range of T_1 and T_2 in biological tissue is known and determines also the measurement parameters. Alternatively,

the training parameter values could be drawn from a given probability distribution, if such
info

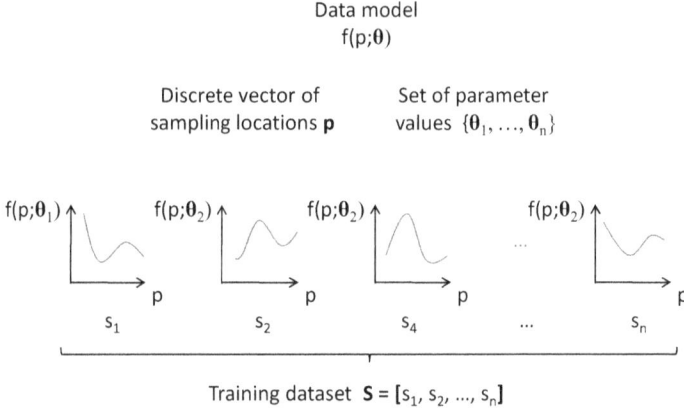

Figure 5.2. Construction of a training data set for a model-based sparsifying transform. A
set of general signal prototypes is obtained by evaluating the model at the sampling locations
$\mathbf{p}$ for a large set of parameter values $\boldsymbol{\theta}_j$.

5.3   Model-based reconstruction using PCA

5.3.1   Sparsity: Model-based Transform

One possible way to define a model-based sparsifying transform is to use the principal component analysis (PCA). PCA is a classical tool for data analysis, visualization and compression [136]. It represents the data as a linear combination of the vectors called principal components, corresponding to orthogonal directions maximizing the variance in the data. Dimensionality reduction is achieved by considering only the principal components corresponding to
the largest eigenvalues. Often just a few principal components are necessary to achieve a good
signal approximation. Also, for a linear approximation with M out of N vectors and multivari-
ate Gaussian statistics, the PCA basis is the transform that shows the minimal approximation
error among all orthogonal bases [42].

The model-based sparsifying transform is obtained as follows. Training data $\mathbf{S}$ are generated
as described in section 5.2. Next the singular value decomposition (SVD) of the correlation
matrix $\mathbf{R} = \mathbf{SS}^H$ is computed.

$$\mathbf{R} = \mathbf{SS}^H = \mathbf{U\Sigma U}^H \tag{5.1}$$

The matrix $\mathbf{U}^H$, taken from the singular value decomposition of the correlation matrix, defines the PCA transform. A multiplication with $\mathbf{U}^H$ rotates the data into a new coordinate system, such that the most significant information is contained in the first few dimensions. Dimensionality reduction could be achieved by approximating the signal in these few dimensions and cropping all the rest. The full matrix $\mathbf{U}^H$, without cropping, is an orthogonal linear operator which achieves a sparse representation of the training set and also of any other signal, described by the model in the given parameter range.

5.3.2 Sampling and Incoherence

The sampling pattern considered in this chapter is illustrated in Fig. 5.1b. Random undersampling in k_y–p (on a Cartesian grid) is performed with variable sampling density in k_y, taking into account that most energy of MR images is concentrated in the low frequencies, and with uniform density in p. This choice is mainly motivated by its compatibility with multi-echo acquisition sequences. Alternatively, the sampling density in p can be adapted to the signal distribution. Incoherence plays an important role in CS and sparse signal approximation. Low coherence guarantees that sparse recovery algorithms can exactly recover any sufficiently sparse signal and that this solution is unique.

The coherence of the PCA transform can be assessed by means of the transform point spread function ($TPSF$) (Eq.(3.26)). The PCA transform is a 1D transform along the temporal direction and the measurement is represented by a 2D or 3D undersampled Fourier transform applied in the spatial directions

$$TPSF(i,j) = \mathbf{e}_j \mathbf{U}^H \mathbf{F}_u^H \mathbf{F}_u \mathbf{U} \mathbf{e}_i. \qquad (5.2)$$

Here $\mathbf{e}_j$ is a vector in the sparsifying transform domain with a single non-zero element of 1 at position j, $\mathbf{U}^H$ and $\mathbf{F}_u$ denote the PCA transform and the undersampled Fourier transform operators. An example of the aliasing pattern for a given sampling pattern and PCA transform is shown in Fig. 5.3. Figures 5.3(a) and (b) show the aliasing in the PCA coefficients along the parameter direction (a) and along the phase encoding direction (b). The example is given for a single PCA coefficient placed in the center of the image. For the same sampling pattern, the aliasing in the image domain is significantly higher as seen in 5.3 (c) and (d).

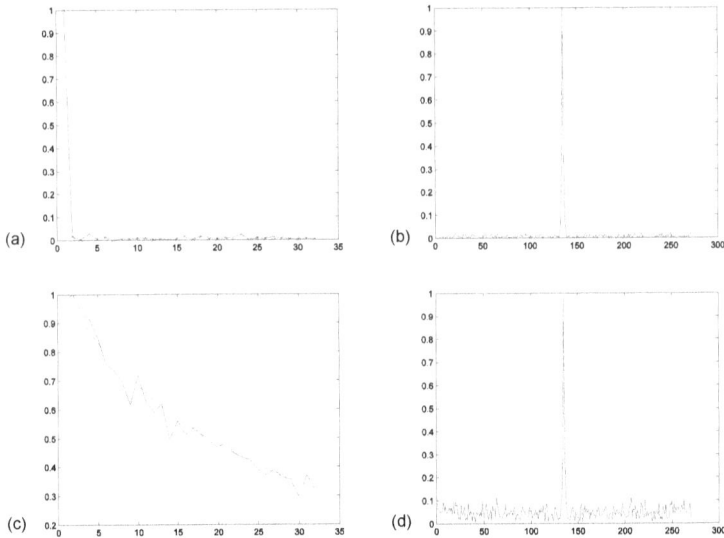

Figure 5.3. Coherence of the PCA transform. The aliasing pattern for random undersampling in the k_y-p domain is shown in the PCA transformed data in the parameter direction (**a**) and in the phase encoding direction (**b**). The aliasing pattern in the image series is shown in the parameter direction (**c**) and in the phase encoding direction (**d**). The red line in (**c**) is the original signal, corresponding to a single PCA coefficient. Due to random undersampling in the parameter direction the aliasing in the PCA domain is significantly decreased compared to the image domain.

5.4 Model-based reconstruction using overcomplete dictionaries

5.4.1 Sparsity: Model-based Transform

Most commonly, orthonormal bases are applied as sparsifying transforms for CS. However, representing a signal with respect to an overcomplete dictionary adds more flexibility in the signal representation and could significantly improve sparsity. A dictionary is a collection of discrete-time signal prototypes (atoms) and is overcomplete if the number of atoms is greater than the signal dimensionality. Large data-adapted dictionaries allow for accurate data description with just a few atoms and in this way achieve much sparser representations compared to orthonormal bases.

Mallat et. al [55] compare signal decomposition in an orthonormal basis and in an overcomplete dictionary to a text written with a small and large vocabulary. While a small vocabulary might be sufficient to express an idea, it requires the use of large sentences for missing words. Similarly, large data-adapted dictionaries allow for accurate data description with just a few atoms and in this way achieve much more compact representations compared to orthonormal bases.

Finding an overcomplete dictionary that sparsely describes the signal is not a trivial task. One possibility is to use a pre-specified set of functions to form a dictionary, e.g by concatenating vectors of different bases such as wavelets, curvelets, delta pulses, etc. In this way, different signal characteristics like edges or point-like singularities could be sparsely described by the atoms from different bases. Choosing a pre-specified transform matrix is appealing because it is simpler. Also, in many cases it leads to simple and fast algorithms for the evaluation of the sparse representation. This is for instance the case for overcomplete wavelets, curvelets, contourlets, short-time-Fourier transforms, and more. Typically, tight frames are preferred that can easily be pseudo-inverted. Better results can be obtained if the dictionary is adapted to a given set of signal examples.

An overcomplete dictionary that sparsely represents the training data can be designed by the K-SVD method proposed by Aharon et al. [137]. The K-SVD algorithm works iteratively, applying two steps in each iteration:

1. in the sparse coding step, the dictionary $\mathbf{D}$ is fixed, and a sparse representation with respect to that dictionary is obtained;

2. in the dictionary update step, the dictionary columns are updated, one column at a time to minimize the approximation error of the training data.

The learned dictionary is optimized for a signal approximation with at most K atoms. The value of K is chosen as small as possible, such that the approximation error in the learned dictionary is below a given threshold, e.g. 10^{-5}. Finding a signal representation of a signal $\mathbf{x}$ with respect to a dictionary $\mathbf{D}$ with at most K coefficients requires solving the problem:

$$\text{minimize } \|\mathbf{x} - \mathbf{Dz}\|_2 \text{, subject to } \|\mathbf{z}\|_0 \leq K. \tag{5.3}$$

This problem is solved at each iteration of the K-SVD algorithm, which motivates the use of efficient algorithms such as the orthogonal matching pursuit (OMP) [78].

The model-based dictionary is applied in the parameter - encoding dimension p. However, each one-dimensional signal in the parameter dimension is related to the complete k-p dataset, requiring joint estimation of the complete dataset. Further sparsity in the image domain can be imposed by applying wavelets or finite differences.

5.4.2   Sampling and incoherence

To obtain a unique sparse representation the dictionary $\mathbf{D}$ has to be incoherent. If the dictionary $\mathbf{D}$ is coherent, the matrix $\mathbf{A} = \mathbf{\Phi D}$ mapping the sparse coefficients $\mathbf{z}$ to the measurement vector $\mathbf{y}$, $\mathbf{y} = \mathbf{Az}$ will also be coherent, which is compromising the CS reconstruction of the sparse representation. Therefore, it is natural to require that the complete matrix $\mathbf{A} = \mathbf{\Phi D}$ is incoherent. However, if we are only interested in the image $\mathbf{x}$ and not in its sparse representation $\mathbf{z}$, the coherence of the dictionary might not be necessary.

If two columns of the dictionary D are closely correlated it will be impossible in general to distinguish if the signal energy is coming from the one or the other. For example, if two atoms of the dictionary are identical, a signal $\mathbf{x} = \mathbf{Dz}$ can be explained with the first or the second or any linear combination of the two atoms. Thus, the sparse representation of the vector $\mathbf{x}$ with respect to the dictionary $\mathbf{D}$ is not unique. However, finding any of these possible representations will lead back to the signal of interest $\mathbf{x} = \mathbf{Dz}$.

In the considered application of MR parameter mapping, the measurement matrix $\mathbf{F}_u$ (related to the sampling in k–p space) is incoherent as it has been shown in Fig. 5.3. The proposed sampling pattern in k–p space results in noise-like artifacts in both the image and the parameter dimensions, which can be removed in the reconstruction. The model-based dictionary may have high coherence, caused by the correlations between signals with different parameters values. However, the large correlation between columns in $\mathbf{D}$ does not impose a problem. Although that makes it impossible to obtain a unique reconstruction of the coefficient vectors $\mathbf{z}$, which is not the goal, it does not compromise the estimation of the desired vector $\mathbf{x}$. As it will be shown in the experiments, the model-based dictionary allows obtaining a very accurate signal approximation with just a few atoms for signals drawn from the data model. Because of the high redundancy, also signals with parameter values not included in the training set are described very sparsely. On the other hand, the dictionary is very discriminative and gives a very poor representation of signals unrelated to the model as well as noise. This enables efficient reduction of the incoherent artifacts in the image series in the reconstruction.

5.5   Reconstruction

A POCS algorithm is chosen for the reconstruction for its simplicity. The algorithm is described here for the case of sparse representation in an overcompe dictionary. It can be easily modified for the PCA transform.

Given a measurement vector $\mathbf{y}$ in k–p space, the goal is to reconstruct the image series $\mathbf{x}$, consisting of L images $\mathbf{x}_l$ at parameter - encoding values p_l, $l = 1, ..., L$. The signal in the parameter dimension at voxel n is denoted with $\mathbf{x}_n$, where $n = 1, ..., N$, and N is the number of voxels.

The sparsity parameter K in the dictionary representation is estimated during the dictionary training phase and is fixed. The K-term estimate is obtained using OMP. The complete data $\mathbf{x}$ are jointly reconstructed, applying the following iterative procedure:

Set $\mathbf{y}^{(0)} = \mathbf{y}$, $\mathbf{x}^{(0)} = \mathbf{0}$. For iteration i:

1. Apply $\mathbf{x}_l^{(i)} = \mathcal{F}_u^H \mathbf{y}_l^{(i-1)}$ for $l = 1, .., L$

2. Compute the K-term estimate $\mathbf{x}_n^{(i)} = \mathbf{D}\mathbf{z}_n^{(i)}$, $||\mathbf{z}_n^{(i)}||_0 = K$, $n = 1, ..., N$

3. Compute $\mathbf{y}_l^{(i)} = \mathcal{F}_u \mathbf{x}_l^{(i)}$ for $l = 1, .., L$ and insert the measured data at the sampling locations $\mathbf{y}^{(i)} = \mathbf{y}|_{acq}$

4. Repeat steps 1-3 until the change of energy in $\mathbf{x}$ gets smaller than a given threshold $\frac{||\mathbf{x}^{(i)} - \mathbf{x}^{(i-1)}||}{||\mathbf{x}^{(i)}||} < \epsilon$

Here $\mathcal{F}_u$ is the undersampled Fourier operator and H denotes the Hermitian conjugate. The algorithm can also be used with the PCA transform. In this case, the OMP in step 2 can be replaced by soft thresholding.

Additional sparsity in the images can be exploited, for instance, by including the following step, denoted as

2'. Compute $\mathbf{x}_l^{(i)} = \mathbf{\Psi}^{-1}\mathcal{T}(\mathbf{\Psi}\mathbf{x}_l^{(i)}, t_l)$, $l = 1, ..., L$, where $\mathcal{T}$ is the soft thresholding operation and $\mathbf{\Psi}$ is a wavelet transform.

The extended algorithm applies steps 2 and 2' alternately during the iterations. The threshold t is determined according to estimation of the signal sparsity.

To evaluate the proposed model-based sparsifying transforms, the following reconstruction variants were studied:

A. Apply the model-based PCA transform in the parameter-encoding dimension and wavelets (Daubechies 4) on the images;

B. Apply only the PCA transform in the parameter-encoding dimension;

C. Apply the model-based dictionary in the parameter-encoding dimension and wavelets (Daubechies 4) on the images;

D. Apply only the dictionary in the parameter-encoding dimension;

E. Apply wavelets on the images and in the parameter-encoding dimension.

Variants **A** and **C** are the recommended approaches for application of the two model-based transform. Variants **B** and **D** show the performance of each model-based transform used alone. Variant **E** is the classical approach, using a general wavelet transform instead of model-based transform and is used as a reference.

5.6   Application to T_1 and T_2 mapping

5.6.1   Data Model

In this work, model-based CS reconstruction is applied to accelerate T_1 and T_2 measurements. The detectable MR signal M in these and some other measurements (e.g. diffusion) can be generalized to the exponential model

$$M(p) = \alpha + \beta \exp(-p/\tau), \tag{5.4}$$

where τ denotes the tissue parameter in question and α and β are complex parameters, which are also estimated in the fit. For estimating these parameters spatially resolved, k-space data need to be acquired at several different values of the acquisition parameter p. The sampling locations of p are determined by the expected range of the relaxation parameters. Uniform sampling with p_{max} about two times the target value of τ is a common choice.

5.6.2   Simulations

To demonstrate the ability of the model-based transforms to sparsely represent data and account for the effects of noise, a computer model was implemented mimicking a T_2 mapping experiment. The simulated phantom data shown in Fig. 5.4 consisted of 32 images with echo time spacing of 12.5 ms, matrix size of 256×256, containing five compartments with different T_2 values (12 – 250 ms). Gaussian noise with $\sigma = 0.02$ (SNR = 50) was added to simulate noisy data.

A training set of 1000 exponentials was generated with decay coefficients uniformly distributed between 1 and 300 ms. The training data were used to determine a PCA transform $\mathbf{U}^H$ and an overcomplete dictionary $\mathbf{D}$. A dictionary with 100 atoms was learned using K-SVD, optimized for a support $K = 3$. The T_2 values of the phantom data were not contained in the training set. A signal approximation with respect to the two model-based transforms was obtained for different numbers of sparse coefficients. The signal approximation with respect to the PCA transform was obtained by thresholding. The approximation with respect to the dictionary was obtained using OMP. The normalized RMS error was used as a quality measure of the approximation.

$$NRMSE = \sqrt{\frac{\sum_{i=1}^{N} |x_i - o_i|^2}{\sum_{i=1}^{N} |o_i|^2}} \tag{5.5}$$

where x_i denotes the i-th voxel of the approximated images and o_i the corresponding voxel in the original images. The sum runs over the entire image series.

The simulation data were undersampled with various reduction factors (2 to 8) and reconstructed with each of the reconstruction variants, described above. Parameter maps were obtained from the set of images on a voxel-by-voxel basis using the Levenberg-Marquardt al-

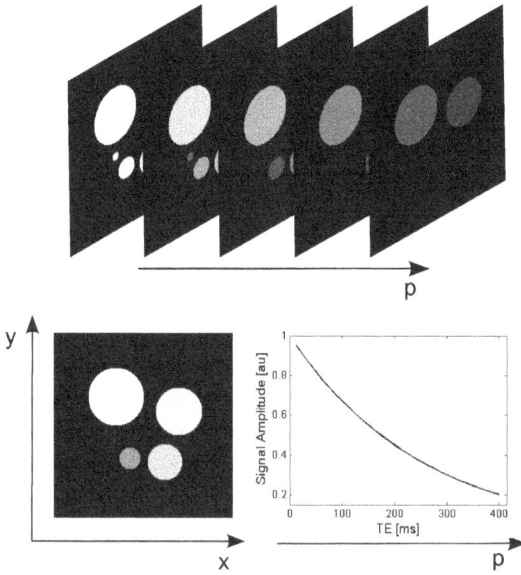

Figure 5.4. The simulation model of T_2 data. A simple numerical phantom was generated consisting of five compartments with different time constants (12 – 250 ms). In total, 32 images were generated along the parameter dimension.

gorithm.

5.6.3 Measurements

The reconstruction technique described above was further demonstrated for the application of T_1 and T_2 mapping *in vivo*. T_1 and T_2 data in the brain were acquired in four healthy volunteers. Measurements were performed on a 1.5T clinical scanner.

For T_1 mapping, inversion recovery data were acquired with a Look-Locker sequence including a correction for apparent T_1 values. The following parameters were used for the measurement: 40 inversion times with increment $\Delta T_i = 72$ ms, inversion repetition time 3 s, FOV 250×250 mm^2, 7 mm slice thickness, 224×224 matrix. Data at each inversion time were acquired with a segmented gradient echo sequence (TE = 1.9 ms, TR = 3.8 ms, flip angle 10°).

For T_2 mapping, multi-spin-echo measurements were performed with the following parameters: 32 echoes, 5 ms echo spacing, TR = 1 s, FOV 250×250 mm^2, 6 mm slice thickness, 256×256 matrix.

The datasets were undersampled retrospectively with reduction factors of 2, 4, 6, and 8 for the T_1-dataset and 2, 3, 4, and 5 for the T_2-dataset. The undersampled data were reconstructed with each of the five variants described above. A PCA transform and a dictionary consisting of 100 atoms were trained for each model. The training dataset for the T_1 model consisted of

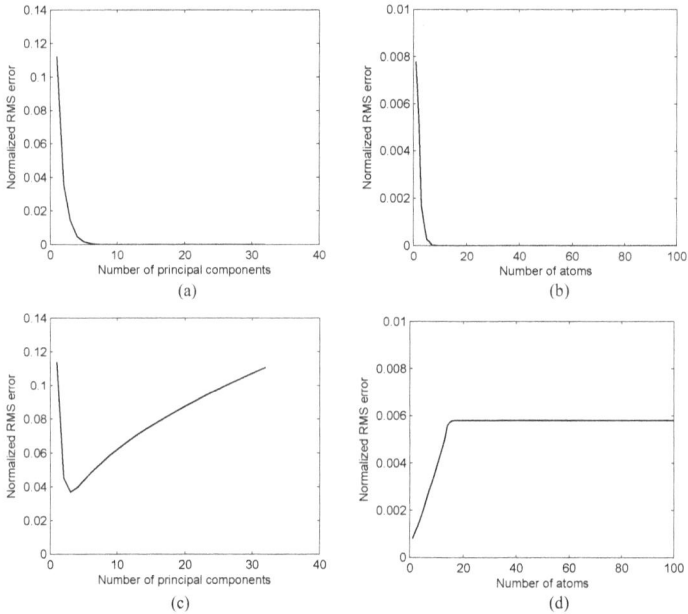

Figure 5.5. Approximation error of the model-based transforms. The NRMSE is plotted as a function of the number of principal components ((**a**), (**c**)) and dictionary atoms ((**b**), (**d**)) used in the approximation. Both transforms achieve a very good signal approximation of noiseless data with few coefficients (**a**), (**b**). Applied to noisy data, most of the signal is contained in the first few coefficients and the noise is (partly) approximated by adding further coefficients (**c**), (**d**). The dictionary representation results in much smaller error in both the noiseless and the noisy case.

2500 exponentials corresponding to apparent T_1s between 0.2 and 500 ms. The dataset for the T_2 model consisted of 1000 exponentials with decay constants between 1 and 300 ms.

Parameter maps were obtained from the reconstructed image series and compared to the true parameter map. The reconstructed image series and the resulting maps were compared to the full sampling case. To assess the reconstruction quality, the NRMSE was calculated for the reconstructed image series and the corresponding parameter maps.

5.7   Results

5.7.1   Simulations

The approximation error as a function of the number of coefficients in the sparsifying transform (PCA and dictionary) is shown in Fig. 5.5. In the noiseless case, both transforms give a very accurate approximation with two or three coefficients and an exact signal representation

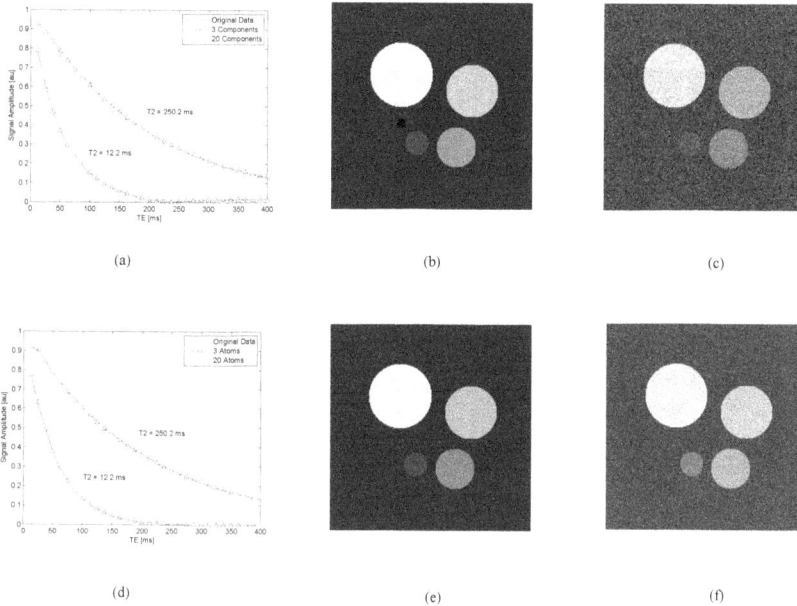

(a)

(b)

(c)

(d)

(e)

(f)

Figure 5.6. Signal approximation of noisy data with PCA transform (top) and model-adapted dictionary (bottom). The signal in the temporal dimension and its approximation with three and twenty coefficients for low and high T_2 values is shown in (a) and (d). The corresponding images for TE = 250 ms are shown in (b) and (e) for an approximation with three coefficients and (c) and (f) with twenty coefficients, for the PCA and the dictionary, respectively.

with less than 10 coefficients (Fig. 5.5 (a, b)). The approximation error using the model-adapted dictionary is much smaller compared with the error using the PCA transform (note the difference in the scales of the NRMSE in Fig. 5.5).

In the presence of noise, the PCA transform approximates most of the exponential signal in the first two or three coefficients, and adding more components essentially adds only noise (Fig. 5.5 (c)). The dictionary is very discriminative to noise. With increasing number of atoms some of the noise is approximated, however, a large portion is discarded (Fig. 5.5 (d)). In both cases the dictionary gives a much more accurate representation of the original signal.

The denoising effect of the sparse approximations is illustrated in Fig. 5.6. Figures 5.6 (a) and (d) show the signal approximation in the parameter direction for the two sparsifying transforms using three and twenty coefficients compared to the original signal. The signal in the parameter dimension is given for a short and a long T_2 value. The approximation with three coefficients already gives a good approximation of the exponential decay. Adding more coefficients approximates also some of the noise. Figures 5.6 (b), (c), (e), and (f) show the signal approximation in the image domain for a given echo time (TE = 250 ms). Since in

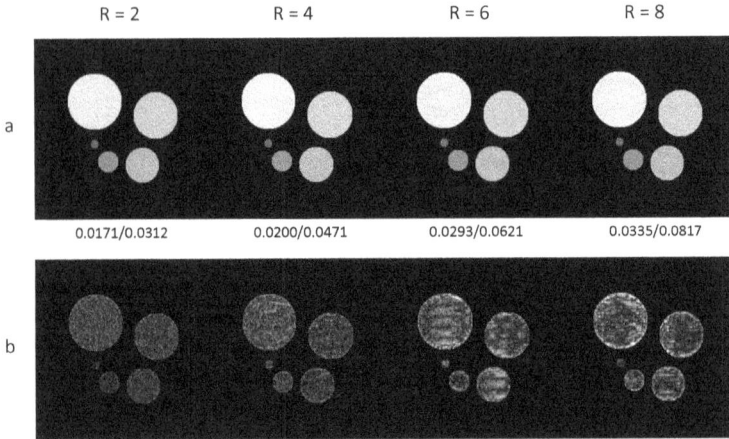

Figure 5.7. T_2 parameter map CS reconstruction of simulated noisy data using a PCA model-based transform. The maps obtained from reconstruction variant **A** are shown in **(a)** for different undersampling factors. For comparison, the NRMSE with respect to the ideal map for reconstruction variants **A** (PCA and wavelets) and **B** (PCA only) is indicated below the maps. The difference images between the maps shown in **(a)** and the ideal map are shown in **(b)**.

CS reconstruction small coefficients are penalized, it is expected that there will be a denoising effect in the reconstructed image series.

In the following figures, the images from the undersampling experiments for the two recommended reconstruction variants **A** and **C** are shown.

Figures 5.7 and 5.8 show the maps obtained from the CS reconstructed image series of the simulation dataset. Figure 5.7 shows the maps obtained using the PCA transform and wavelets (variant **A**). The maps obtained with variant **B** show larger error. This can be seen in the NRMSE with respect to the ideal map, which is indicated for reconstruction variants **A** and **B** below each map. Figure 5.8 shows the maps obtained using the dictionary and wavelets (variant **C**). The NRMSE for reconstruction variants **C**, **D** and **E** is given for each reduction factor.

Accurate parameter maps were obtained for all reduction factors. The error for a reduction factor of 6 in reconstruction variant **C** (Fig. 5.8) and a reduction factor 2 in reconstruction variant **A** (Fig. 5.7) is about the same as for the map, obtained from 32 fully sampled echoes ($NRMSE = 0.0179$) as a consequence of the finite SNR. The denoising effect of the reconstruction results in decreased errors for lower reduction factors. With increasing reduction factor the error in the maps changes from noise-like to localized (artifacts). Reconstruction variant **C** gives the best results in both NRMSE and visual quality for all reduction factors.

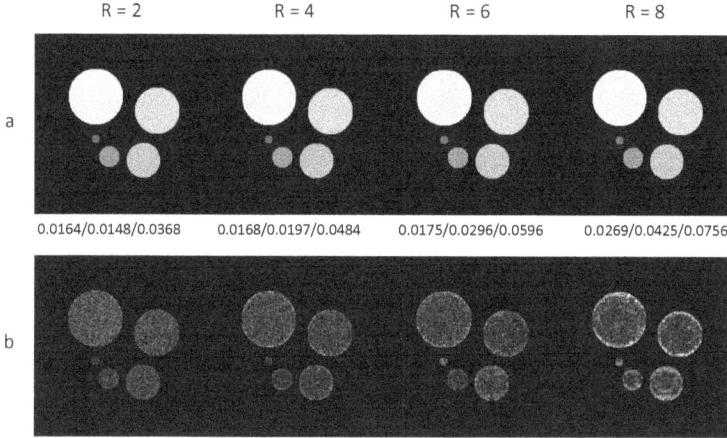

Figure 5.8. T_2 parameter map CS reconstruction of simulated noisy data using a model-based dictionary. The maps obtained from image series reconstructed with the proposed model-based reconstruction (reconstruction variant **C**) are shown for different undersampling factors in **(a)**. For comparison, the NRMSE with respect to the ideal map for reconstruction variants **C** (dictionary and wavelets), **D** (dictionary only) and **E** (wavelets in all directions) is given below the maps. Note that a conventional parameter mapping reconstruction using fully sampled data results in a NRMSE of 0.0179 because of the finite SNR in the data. The corresponding error maps are shown in **(b)**.

5.7.2 Measurements

Figures 5.9 and 5.10 show selected results from the *in vivo* T_1 mapping experiments. A single image picked from the acquired image series is shown for full Nyquist sampling (R= 1) and for CS reconstruction with reduction factors of 2 to 8 in (a). As expected, a slight denoising is observed in the CS reconstructed images. All aliasing artifacts in the images, resulting from the undersampling, could be removed for a reduction factor up to 6 for the dictionary and up to 4 for the PCA transform. For higher reduction factors some residual aliasing as well as blurring is observed in the reconstructed images. The resulting T_1 maps are shown in Figs. 5.9 (b) and 5.10 (b). The quality of the maps corresponds well to the quality of the image series. The model-based dictionary (variant **C**) results in slightly better reconstruction than variant **A**.

Results from the T_2 mapping experiments are shown in Figs. 5.11 and 5.12. Accurate reconstruction was achieved for data reduction factors up to 4. For higher reduction factors, the image quality is visibly decreased.

Also here, the model-based CS reconstruction results in maps very close to the full sampling map. Variants **A** and **C** show very similar results with a slight advantage for variant **C**.

Images for all five reconstruction variants are shown in Fig. 5.13 for the example of R = 3.

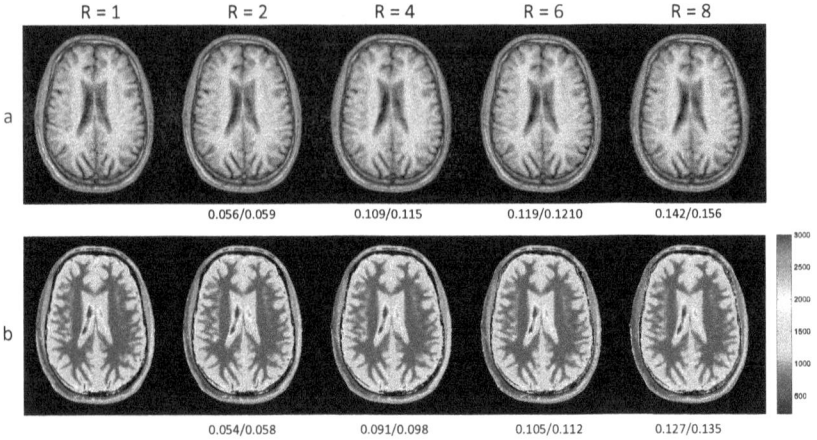

Figure 5.9. CS reconstruction of T_1 mapping data applying a model-based PCA transform. (a) The image for TI = 1.65 s and full sampling (R=1), as well as CS reconstruction with various reduction factors. (b) the resulting T_1 maps do not show any visible differences compared to the reference map up to a reduction factor of 6. The normalized RMS error with respect to the fully sampled map is given below each image. The color-coding bar indicates the T_1 times in ms.

The reconstruction variants using only a PCA transform in the parameter direction (variant **B**) and wavelets in the image and parameter direction (variant **E**) show significant artifacts already at R = 3. The images reconstructed with the dictionary only (variant **D**) have a good image quality. They appear more grainy, compared to the case when wavelets in the image domain are applied additionally (variant **C**).

The reconstruction variant **C**, applying learned dictionary in the para- meter-encoding dimension and wavelets in the image dimension, shows the smallest NRMSE in all experiments. Applying the dictionary alone results in similar reconstruction quality for most of the cases. Significant improvement of using both transforms together has only been achieved in the phantom experiments. In all experiments, the standard reconstruction (variant **E**) shows artifacts for a reduction factors of 3 and higher. The number of required iterations was between 6 and 35 depending on the reduction factor. The computation time for one iteration was about 29s for a $256 \times 256 \times 32$ matrix (Matlab, 2.2GHz CPU).

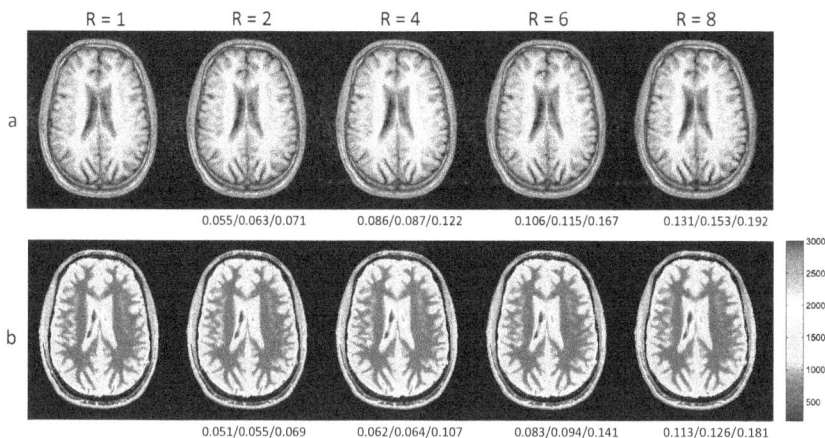

Figure 5.10. CS reconstruction of T_1 mapping data applying a model-based dictionary. **(a)** Images for TI = 1.65 s and full sampling (R = 1) and CS reconstructions with various reduction factors (R = 2, ..., 8). Slight denoising is observed in the CS-reconstructed images. **(b)**The resulting T_1 maps do not show any visible differences compared to the reference map up to a reduction factor of 6. The NRMSE with respect to the fully sampled image/map is given below each image/map for the reconstruction cases **C/D/E**. The color-coding bar indicates the T_1 times in ms.

5.8 Discussion

Prior knowledge of the signal model was incorporated in the CS reconstruction by applying a sparsifying transform, learned from the data model. Two different transforms were considered which sparsify the data in the parameter direction: an orthonormal transform, obtained by PCA, and an overcomplete dictionary. The model-based transforms were applied in the CS reconstruction of undersampled T_1- and T_2-mapping data, achieving accurate reconstructions with acceleration factors of about $4-6$. The overcomplete dictionary results in sparser data representation and leads to better CS reconstructions compared to the PCA transform, when these transforms are used alone. Enforcing additional sparsity in the wavelet domain can further improve the reconstruction. This improvement is significant mostly for the PCA transform, while for the dictionary the improvement is noticeable only for images with very sparse wavelet representation.

The best reconstruction in the numerical phantom experiments was obtained applying the overcomplete dictionary and wavelets. Variant **C** also yielded very good results in the in vivo

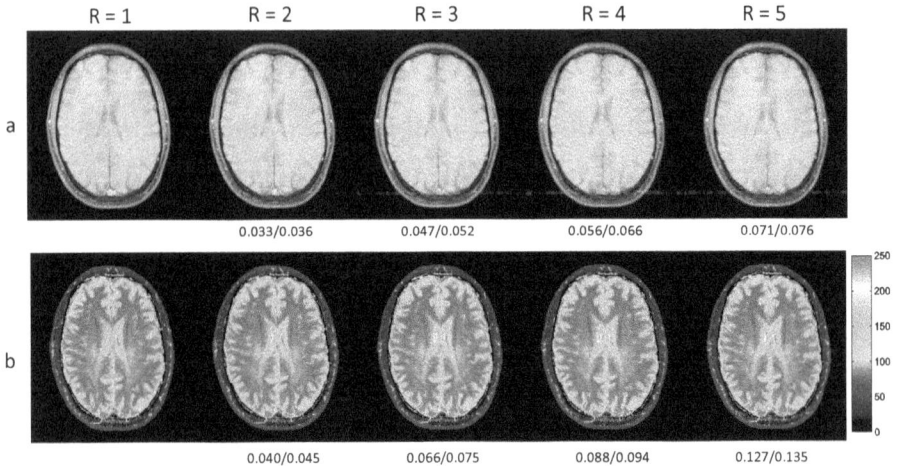

Figure 5.11. CS reconstruction of T_2 mapping data with PCA transform. **(a)** Image for TE = 20 ms and full sampling (R = 1) and CS reconstructions with reduction factors 2 to 5. b) The corresponding T_2 maps. The color-coding bar indicates the T_2 times in ms. The NRMSE error for reconstruction variants **A** (PCA and wavelets) and **B** (PCA only) is given for each undersampling factor.

experiments. However, the results aobtained with the PCA transform and wavelets **A** are also very similar. The achievable reduction factors may vary for different datasets depending on data compressibility, data size, sampling pattern, SNR or potentially deviations from the model.

The sparsity of the signal representation with respect to an overcomplete dictionary depends on the training data and on the dictionary size. Generally, the sparsity can be improved by increasing the dictionary size but this also increases the computational burden and the dictionary coherence. Although the model-based dictionary may have high coherence, a surprisingly good sparse signal approximation was obtained with OMP, and as a consequence a good CS reconstruction. Similar observations have been reported in a recent work by Wright et al. [138], showing clear advantage of coherent dictionaries in the signal recovery from randomly corrupted images. A heuristic explanation of this may be that the signal of interest spans a small portion of the space and the learned dictionary represents that space well, while rejecting signals outside of it. One can think of the orthonormal PCA transform as an incoherent dictionary. The orthogonality of the PCA transform assures that the signal representation in this transform domain is unique. It has also been shown that random sampling in the k-p space leads to reduced coherence in the PCA transformed domain compared to the image domain, because it makes use of the additional parameter dimension p, while the images in the image series are

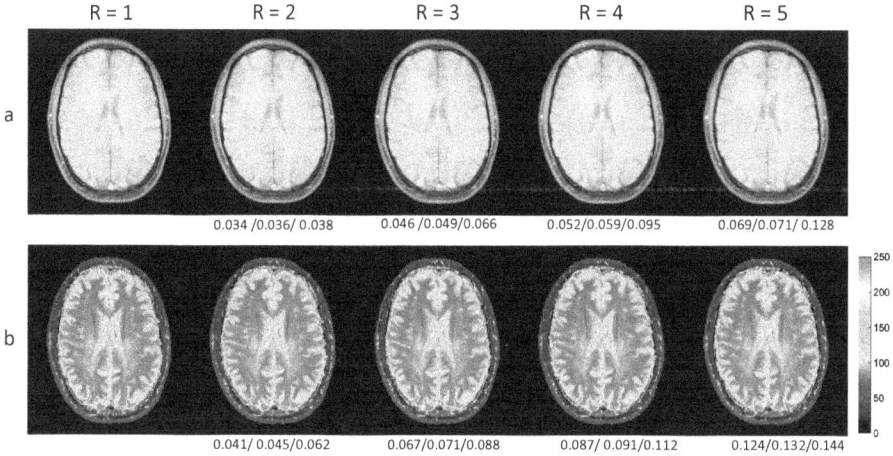

Figure 5.12. CS reconstruction of T_2 mapping data with model-based dictionary. **(a)** Image for TE = 20 ms and full sampling (R = 1) and CS reconstructions with reduction factors 2 to 5. **(b)** The corresponding T_2 maps. The color-coding bar indicates the T_2 times in ms. The NRMSE error for the three reconstruction variants **C** (dictionary and wavelets), **D** (dictionary only) and **E** (wavelets in the image and the parameter directions) is given for each undersampling factor.

decoupled.

In a dictionary with infinitely many atoms, the signal can be ultimately represented by a single atom. This is equivalent to fitting the signal to the model. Thus, another possible reconstruction approach would be to fit the undersampled data to the model at each iteration and subtract the artifacts from the resulting signal approximation. Another related approach would be to combine the CS reconstruction with a nonlinear inversion approach like the one presented in [139], jointly estimating the images and the parameter map. These two approaches could be an interesting alternative to the one proposed here, however they involve nonlinear sparsifying transforms or nonlinear measurements, which are not considered in the existing CS theory. Furthermore, there might be difficulties regarding the numerical stability due to the nonlinearity and multiple local minima as well as increased computational complexity.

In practice, the tissue in each voxel is not always homogeneous, and tissues with different parameters could contribute to the signal by means of partial volume effects. Multi-exponential fits can be applied in this case to decrease errors due to partial volume effects and to characterize multi-compartmental relaxation curves [140]. Multi-exponential analysis have been applied to identify and characterize multiple water compartments in normal and pathologic tissue in different anatomies [141–146]. Some of these works consider measurements of T_2 spectra/distributions in tissue acquiring several thousand echoes [144–146]. The presented model-

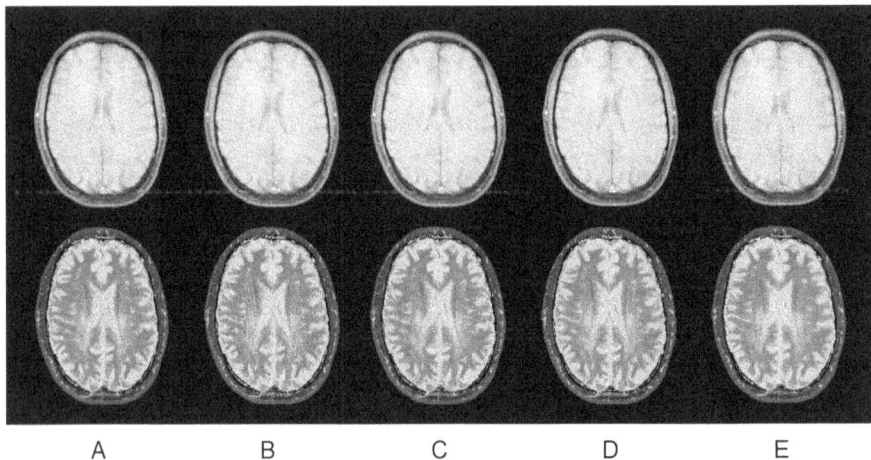

Figure 5.13. Comparison of CS reconstructions of T_2 mapping data with different sparsifying transforms. T_2 mapping data with an undersampling factor of three is shown for all considered reconstruction variants **A** (PCA transform and wavelets), **B** (PCA transform only), **C** (learned dictionary and wavelets), **D** (learned dictionary only), and **E** (wavelets in the temporal and image domain). An image for TE = 20 ms (top) and the T_2 map (bottom) are shown for all reconstruction variants.

based transforms do not restrict the signal to a single exponential. In fact, the reconstructed signal is a linear combination of multiple exponentials, so the reconstruction is also compatible with a multi-exponential fit.

Model-based CS reconstruction was demonstrated here for the applications of accelerated T_1 and T_2 mapping in the brain. However, there are also other applications, in which the same approach is applicable. The signal model in diffusion measurements is also exponential, equivalent to the T_2 mapping model, so the same reconstruction is also applicable for diffusion measurements. One could also apply the model-based transforms for more complex MR tissue signal models, as for instance perfusion.

Several other methods exist to speed up sampling in MRI. Such methods, for instance, are partial k-space sampling, exploiting the conjugate symmetry of the Fourier transform of real images, and parallel imaging. A combination with these methods could potentially allow even higher data reduction and thus higher acceleration factors.

CHAPTER SIX

CS FOR CHEMICAL SHIFT-BASED
WATER-FAT SEPARATION

The devil has put a penalty on all things we enjoy in life. Either we suffer in health or we suffer in soul or we get fat.

— ALBERT EINSTEIN

Multi-echo chemical shift-based water-fat separation methods allow for uniform fat suppression in the presence of main field inhomogeneities. However, these methods require additional scan time for chemical shift encoding. This chapter presents a method for water-fat separation from undersampled data (CS-WF), which combines compressed sensing and chemical shift-based water-fat separation. Undersampling is applied in k-space and in the chemical shift encoding dimension to reduce the total scan time. The method can reconstruct high quality water and fat images in 2D and 3D imaging from highly undersampled data. As an extension, multi-peak fat spectral models are incorporated into the CS-WF reconstruction to improve the water-fat separation quality. In 3D MRI, reduction factors of above three can be achieved, thus fully compensating the additional time needed in triple-echo water-fat imaging. The method is demonstrated on knee and abdominal in vivo data.

Based upon: M. Doneva, P. Börnert, H. Eggers, A. Mertins, J. Pauly, and M. Lustig "Compressed Sensing for Chemical Shift based Water-Fat Separation", *Magn Reson Med 2010*.

6.1   Introduction

I n vivo MR images usually contain signals from several chemical species, of which water and fat are the most prominent ones. Fat often appears rather bright in MR images and may obscure underlying pathology, degrading their diagnostic value. To overcome this problem, reliable fat suppression methods need to be applied. Common fat suppression techniques include fat saturation [147], spectral-spatial water selective excitation [7], and short-TI inversion recovery [116]. However, these techniques have certain limitations such as high sensitivity to B_0 inhomogeneities, RF inhomogeneities, or low SNR.

Water-fat separation methods based on chemical shift-induced phase differences allow for fat suppression in a more robust way, since field inhomogeneities can be estimated from the data and taken into account in the water-fat separation. Early works on chemical shift imaging include the two-point Dixon method [148] and the multi-point spectroscopic approach proposed by Sepponen et al. [149]. Many variations of these multi-point water-fat separation methods have later been derived [150–153], which exploit the potential to correct for field inhomogeneities. Multi-point methods deliver high SNR due to the internal signal averaging in the reconstruction. A further advantage of water-fat separation over other fat suppression techniques is that it delivers a fat image in addition to the water image, which can provide additional diagnostic information [92].

Chemical shift-based water-fat separation methods require the acquisition of two or more images at different echo times, which prolongs the total scan time. The acquisition of several 3D images may take too long to be performed within a single breath-hold, causing inconsistencies between the images at different echo times as well as motion artifacts. To improve the imaging efficiency, multi-echo techniques, measuring a number of echoes after each RF excitation, can be used for chemical shift encoding [154,155]. However, their sampling efficiency might not be sufficient to compensate for the extra time needed. To further decrease the scan time, parallel imaging is often applied [154,156].

In this chapter, a method combining compressed sensing (CS) with water-fat separation is described, which compensates for the additional time needed for chemical shift encoding. CS has previously been applied to accelerate MR image acquisition in different applications [69,98,110]. Incoherent sampling, signal sparsity and a nonlinear, sparsity promoting reconstruction are the key elements of a successful CS reconstruction. Carefully choosing these for a given application is important to obtain good reconstruction performance. In chemical shift imaging, additional subsampling in the chemical shift dimension can be employed, resulting in subsampling a higher dimensional space, and thus improved incoherence. Applying a sparsity constraint in the water and fat images effectively exploits this additional subsampling dimension. In this chapter, an integrated CS water-fat separation is proposed (CS-WF), which simultaneously recovers the missing k-space data and performs water-fat separation.

6.2 Water-Fat Separation

6.2.1 The Signal Model

Chemical shift-based water-fat separation methods are often based on the assumption of known and discrete resonance frequencies for water and fat [148]. The acquisition of multiple images at different echo times allows for recovery of the signal from each species. Denoting the k-space data acquired at echo time t_l with $\mathbf{y}_l$, the total measurement vector is given by concatenating all data in the column vector $\mathbf{y} = [\mathbf{y}_1; ...; \mathbf{y}_L]$. The number of required echo times L depends on the complexity of the applied model. Three-point measurements are considered in this work, from which complex water and fat images and a field inhomogeneity map are obtained.

The k-space data acquired at echo time t_l are described by the model:

$$\mathbf{y}_l = \mathcal{F}\{(\boldsymbol{\rho}_w + \boldsymbol{\rho}_f e^{2\pi i \Delta f t_l}) \cdot e^{2\pi i \phi t_l}\} \tag{6.1}$$

Here $\boldsymbol{\rho}_w$ is the water image, $\boldsymbol{\rho}_f$ is the fat image, Δf is the chemical shift between water and fat, $\boldsymbol{\phi}$ is the field map, and $\mathcal{F}$ is the spatial Fourier transform. The vectors $\boldsymbol{\rho}_w$, $\boldsymbol{\rho}_f$, and $\boldsymbol{\phi}$ are of length N, N being the number of voxels. Grouping all the unknowns together in one column vector $\mathbf{x} = [\boldsymbol{\rho}_w; \boldsymbol{\rho}_f; \boldsymbol{\phi}]$, the signal model can be written in the concise form $\mathbf{y} = g(\mathbf{x})$, where $g()$ is the nonlinear operator mapping the water, fat and field map to the acquired k-space locations.

The goal of the reconstruction is to find $\mathbf{x}$ from the measurements $\mathbf{y}$ according to the given signal model $\mathbf{y} = g(\mathbf{x})$.

6.2.2 Multi-Peak Fat Model

The fat spectrum contains multiple resonance frequencies, which contribute to the measured signal. The relative amplitude of the different fat peaks depends on the MR acquisition parameters and could vary for different sequences. This could lead to incomplete water-fat separation if not taken appropriately into account [157].

The simple single-peak fat model can be extended by considering several dominant peaks in the fat spectrum. Recent studies show that the fat spectrum in in vivo human studies can be considered as spatially invariant [158]. Using the assumption of multi-peak spatially invariant fat spectrum the signal model becomes

$$\mathbf{y}_l = \mathcal{F}\{(\boldsymbol{\rho}_w + \boldsymbol{\rho}_f \sum_{m=1}^{M} \alpha_m e^{2\pi i \Delta f_m t_l}) \cdot e^{2\pi i \phi t_l}\}, \tag{6.2}$$

where the chemical shifts Δf_m for each fat peak are known a priori. The relative amplitudes of the fat peaks α_m with $\sum \alpha_m = 1$ could be obtained in a separate calibration scan or by a self-calibration procedure [157]. This allows the incorporation of multi-peak fat models without increasing the number of echoes.

For simplicity, all derivations to the rest of the paper will be given for the single-peak fat model. The extension to a multi-peak fat model is straightforward, by simply replacing the exponential factor in front of the fat term with the sum of exponentials as shown above.

6.2.3   Water-Fat Separation Methods

In the case of full sampling, the water-fat decomposition problem is separable and can be solved voxel-by-voxel. Denoting the image at echo time t_l with $\mathbf{s}_l = \mathcal{F}^{-1}\{\mathbf{y}_l\}$, a single voxel from the image $\mathbf{s}_l$ with spatial index r can be described by the simplified model

$$\mathbf{s}_l(r) = (\boldsymbol{\rho}_w(r) + \boldsymbol{\rho}_f(r)e^{2\pi i \Delta f t_l})e^{2\pi i \phi(r)t_l} \tag{6.3}$$

Here $\boldsymbol{\rho}_w(r)$, $\boldsymbol{\rho}_f(r)$ and $\phi(r)$ denote the values of the water, fat and field map signals at the corresponding voxel.

The water-fat separation at a voxel with index r can be obtained by minimizing the cost function

$$J(\mathbf{x}(r)) = || \underbrace{\begin{bmatrix} e^{2\pi i \phi(r)t_1} & 0 & 0 \\ 0 & e^{2\pi i \phi(r)t_2} & 0 \\ 0 & 0 & e^{2\pi i \phi(r)t_3} \end{bmatrix}}_{\mathbf{D}(r)} \underbrace{\begin{bmatrix} 1 & e^{2\pi i \Delta f t_1} \\ 1 & e^{2\pi i \Delta f t_2} \\ 1 & e^{2\pi i \Delta f t_3} \end{bmatrix}}_{\mathbf{A}}$$

$$\underbrace{\begin{bmatrix} \boldsymbol{\rho}_w(r) \\ \boldsymbol{\rho}_f(r) \end{bmatrix}}_{\rho(r)} - \mathbf{s}(r)||_2^2 \tag{6.4}$$

where $\mathbf{s}(r) = [\mathbf{s}_1(r), ..., \mathbf{s}_3(r)]^T$, the vector $\boldsymbol{\rho}(r)$ contains the water and fat images at voxel r, $\mathbf{A}$ is the chemical shift mixture matrix, and $\mathbf{D}(r)$ is a diagonal matrix comprising the field inhomogeneity terms. The IDEAL method [152] solves the problem by using a nonlinear least squares estimation, iteratively repeating two steps: field map estimation with fixed $\boldsymbol{\rho}(r)$ and estimation of the water and fat signals with fixed field map. IDEAL gives the maximum likelihood estimate for the water-fat decomposition and allows for arbitrary echo times. A major difficulty in the reconstruction is the estimation of the nonlinear parameter $\phi(r)$, since the cost function is non-convex and has multiple local minima.

In case of water-only or fat-only voxels, there are two equivalent local minima, which presents an inherent ambiguity of the water-fat separation problem. In practice, most of the voxels contain one dominant species, so a voxel-by-voxel solution could lead to errors in the decomposition in some voxels. In the case of constant echo spacing ΔTE the cost function is periodic with period $1/\Delta$TE, which may cause additional difficulty in the case of large field inhomogeneities and long echo spacings.

Spatial smoothness of the field map is commonly imposed as a prior to address this problem. Methods enforcing field map smoothness include filtering the field map [152], applying a region growing algorithm [159], and applying a smoothness constraint in an iterative water-fat separation algorithm [160], among others. In the presence of multiple local minima, descent-based approaches find the closest minimum in the descent direction from the initial value. Therefore, a good initialization is crucial for the success of these algorithms.

A more robust approach is to locate multiple local minima for each voxel and to apply a smoothness constraint to obtain a field map from the possible solutions [161–163]. An exhaustive search through all possible solutions takes prohibitively long. However, different heuristics such as region growing/merging [161, 162] or graph cut algorithms [163] can be applied to find a good solution. Methods for locating the multiple local minima proposed in the past include Golden section search [161] and the algebraic approach proposed in [162]. In the latter approach, the global minimum is obtained for voxels containing both water and fat, and several possible solutions are computed for voxels containing one species only.

In this chapter, a simple method is suggested, which provides an analytical solution and includes all local minima as possible candidates for the field map. The method is related to the one proposed in [162], but allows the computation of all local minima, independent of the number of species in each voxel. To derive this solution, the cost function J is represented in terms of the field map only by replacing the vector $\boldsymbol{\rho}(r)$ with its least squares estimate

$$\tilde{\boldsymbol{\rho}}(r) = \mathbf{A}^{+}\mathbf{D}^{-1}(r)\mathbf{s}(r) \tag{6.5}$$

as described in [157] and make a change of variables:

$$
J(\boldsymbol{\phi}(r)) = \left\| (\mathbf{A}\mathbf{A}^{+} - \mathbf{I}) \begin{bmatrix} 1 & 0 & 0 \\ 0 & e^{-2\pi i\phi(r)(\Delta\mathrm{TE})} & 0 \\ 0 & 0 & e^{-2\pi i\phi(r)(2\Delta\mathrm{TE})} \end{bmatrix} \mathbf{s}(r) \right\|_2^2
$$

$$
= \left\| \mathbf{B} \begin{bmatrix} z^0 \\ z^{-1} \\ z^{-2} \end{bmatrix} \right\|_2^2, \tag{6.6}
$$

where

$$\mathbf{A}^{+} = (\mathbf{A}^{H}\mathbf{A})^{-1}\mathbf{A}^{H} \tag{6.7}$$

is the pseudoinverse of $\mathbf{A}$,

$$\mathbf{B} = (\mathbf{A}\mathbf{A}^{+} - \mathbf{I})\mathrm{diag}(\mathbf{s}(r)), \tag{6.8}$$

with $\mathrm{diag}(\mathbf{s}(r))$ being a diagonal matrix containing the elements of vector $\mathbf{s}(r)$ in its main diagonal. The cost function can be represented as a two-sided polynomial

$$J(\phi(r)) = \sum_{n=-2}^{2} \beta_n z^n, \tag{6.9}$$

where $z = e^{2\pi i \phi \Delta \text{TE}}$ and the coefficients β_n are obtained as a sum of the diagonals of the matrix $\mathbf{B}^H \mathbf{B}$. The computation of the coefficients β_n is shown in Fig. 6.1.

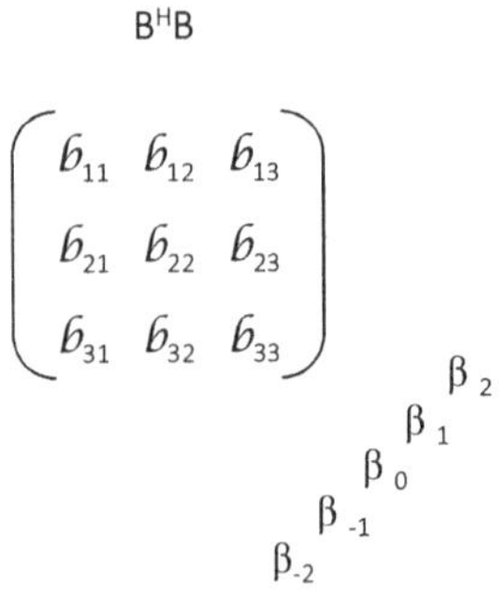

$$\mathsf{B^H B}$$

$$\begin{pmatrix} b_{11} & b_{12} & b_{13} \\ b_{21} & b_{22} & b_{23} \\ b_{31} & b_{32} & b_{33} \end{pmatrix}$$

β_2

β_1

β_0

β_{-1}

β_{-2}

Figure 6.1. The coefficients β_n are computed as sum of the diagonal elements of the matrix $B^H B$ as illustrated in the figure.

The extrema of $J(\phi(r))$ can be found by setting its first derivative to zero

$$G(\phi(r)) = dJ(\phi(r))/d\phi(r) = \sum_{n=-2}^{2} 2\pi i n \Delta \text{TE} \beta_n (e^{2\pi i \phi(r) \Delta \text{TE}})^n = 0. \tag{6.10}$$

The roots of $G(\phi(r))$ are the same as the roots of the one-sided polynomial

$$G^*(\phi(r)) = \sum_{n=0}^{4} \beta_n^* (e^{2\pi i \phi(r) \Delta \text{TE}})^n, \tag{6.11}$$

obtained by multiplying $G(\phi(r))$ with $(e^{2\pi i \phi(r) \Delta \text{TE}})^2$. This is a fourth-order polynomial in terms of $e^{2\pi i \phi(r) \Delta \text{TE}}$, and therefore, $J(\phi(r))$ has four extremal points within a single period, maximally two of which are minima. The minima could be found by checking the second derivative or by probing the neighborhood to determine the type of the extremal point. To obtain the final field map from the multiple local minima, a region growing algorithm was applied, similar to the one described in [161].

6.3 Compressed Sensing for Water-Fat Separation

Compressed sensing [33, 34] allows for signal reconstruction from a small set of random linear measurements by exploiting signal sparsity. Assuming that the signal is sparse in some known transform domain, the sparsest solution agreeing with the given measurements is with very high probability the correct solution.

A naive approach to combine CS and water-fat separation is to perform CS reconstruction on each individual echo data set and do the water-fat separation in a second step. This means that for each individual echo image $\mathbf{s}_l$ the following optimization problem is solved

$$\underset{\mathbf{s}_l}{\operatorname{argmin}} ||\mathbf{\Psi}\mathbf{s}_l||_1, s.t. ||\mathbf{F}_u\mathbf{s}_l - \mathbf{y}_l||_2^2 < \varepsilon, \tag{6.12}$$

where $\mathbf{F}_u$ is the undersampled Fourier matrix corresponding to the applied sampling pattern, $\mathbf{\Psi}$ is the sparsifying transform, and the parameter ε is related to the noise level and the accuracy of the measurement. Subsequently, water-fat separation is applied on the data, recovered by the CS reconstruction. This approach is convenient because the CS reconstruction is performed independently of the water-fat separation. However, it does not use the full potential of CS, because it does not account for correlations between the images at the different echo times. Furthermore, in such decoupled reconstruction the water-fat separation is performed on the data obtained from the CS reconstruction and does not have reference to the original data. Thus, potential errors generated in the CS reconstruction might be amplified in the water-fat separation.

To achieve better data consistency and use the full potential for data undersampling, the CS water-fat separation is formulated as a sparsity constrained nonlinear inverse problem, in which the water and fat images and the field map are the parameters $\mathbf{x} = [\boldsymbol{\rho}_w; \boldsymbol{\rho}_f; \boldsymbol{\phi}]$, and the signal model, mapping $\mathbf{x}$ to the k-space data $\mathbf{y} = g(\mathbf{x})$ (see Eq. [1]), is interpreted as a nonlinear measurement operator. The integrated CS water-fat reconstruction problem can formally be written as:

$$\underset{\mathbf{x}=[\boldsymbol{\rho}_w, \boldsymbol{\rho}_f, \boldsymbol{\phi}]}{\operatorname{argmin}} \{||\mathbf{\Psi}_w\boldsymbol{\rho}_w||_1 + ||\mathbf{\Psi}_f\boldsymbol{\rho}_f||_1\}, s.t. ||g(\mathbf{x}) - \mathbf{y}||_2^2 < \varepsilon, \tag{6.13}$$

where $\mathbf{\Psi}_w$ and $\mathbf{\Psi}_f$ are sparsifying transforms applied to the water and fat images. In other words we are looking for the sparsest solution for the transformed water and fat images $\mathbf{\Psi}_w\boldsymbol{\rho}_w$ and $\mathbf{\Psi}_f\boldsymbol{\rho}_f$, which is consistent with the acquired k-space data and the signal model. CS and water-fat separation are simultaneously performed jointly for all voxels.

6.3.1 Sparsity

Three-point water-fat separation already exploits sparsity in the spectral domain to reduce the number of measurements. This is implied by the signal model, which restricts the signal spectrum to two spectral peaks, one for water and one for fat. This converts the otherwise

spectroscopic problem of water-fat separation to the inverse problem of finding the signal amplitudes for the given frequencies. The (transform) sparsity in the water and fat images could
be used in a CS reconstruction to achieve further data reduction. Similarly to other medical
images, the water and fat images can be sparsified by a finite differences or wavelet transform,
or because most voxels are either fat or water by imposing image sparsity as well. In contrast
to the sequential reconstruction, which exploits the sparsity of three individual echo images,
containing both water and fat, in the integrated reconstruction the data from the three echoes
are combined into the water and fat images, reducing the number of sparse coefficients. Often
the water and fat images contain less structure and can be better sparsified than the combined
echo images.

6.3.2   Sampling

Incoherent sampling is very important in CS. Variable density random sampling of k-space
has been shown to work well for MR CS reconstruction, because most of the signal energy is
concentrated around the k-space origin [69]. In chemical shift imaging, additional random subsampling in the chemical shift encoding dimension can be employed resulting in undersampling
in a higher dimensional $k - \text{TE}$ space and thus in improved incoherence. The signal distribution
in this dimension is quite uniform, so uniform density sampling is a valid choice.

Two possible randomized k-space sampling patterns have been considered: Poisson-disk
sampling [164] and random sampling. Full sampling around the central part of k-space is
applied to account for the image energy distribution. A fully sampled central k-space is also
advantageous, because it can be used for low-resolution field map estimation, as well as for
auto-calibration in case of parallel imaging reconstruction. The two types of sampling are
illustrated in Fig. 6.2. Although an incoherence analysis is difficult because of the nonlinearity
of the model, a simple comparison of the sampling patterns can be made by comparing the
aliasing patterns in the water and fat images caused by the undersampling for a fixed field map.
Fig. 6.2 a) shows the aliasing pattern of the two sampling schemes for a single water voxel. This
is obtained by computing the "point spread function" (PSF) of the system:

$$\hat{\rho} = \mathbf{A}^H \mathbf{D}^H \mathbf{F}_u^H (1/\mathbf{\Theta}) \mathbf{F}_u \mathbf{D} \mathbf{A} \rho. \tag{6.14}$$

Here ρ is a vector of length $2N$ with a single voxel in the water image $\rho(j)$ set to one, $\mathbf{F}_u$ is
the undersampled Fourier operator of the corresponding sampling pattern, $\mathbf{\Theta}$ is the sampling
density, $\mathbf{A}$ and $\mathbf{D}$ are the chemical shift and field map matrices, respectively, defined for the
complete image as block diagonal matrices. The maximum aliasing amplitude $\max_{i \neq j} |\hat{\rho}(i)|$ and
the mean aliasing energy $\frac{1}{N} \sum_{i, i \neq j} \hat{\rho}(i)^H \hat{\rho}(i)$, where N is the total number of voxels, are given
in Fig. 6.2. While both sampling patterns show similar incoherence, the Poisson-disk sampling
has some advantages in terms of better sampling uniformity, which results in decreased aliasing
energy and could also be useful for a later extension to parallel imaging. In the sequential

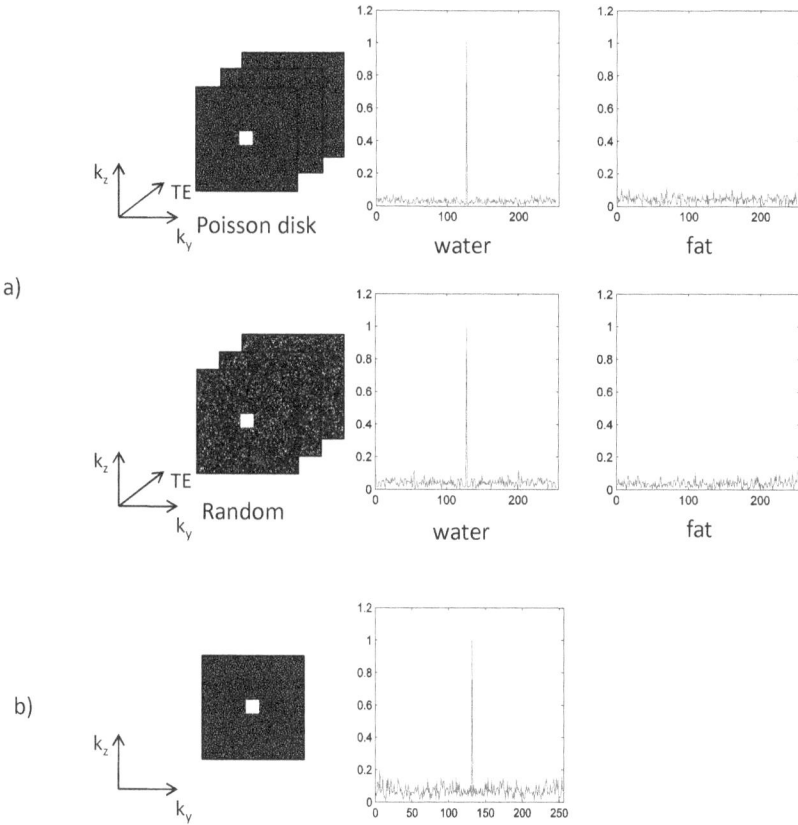

Figure 6.2. Incoherent sampling pattern for CS-WF. a) Incoherent sampling in the phase encoding and temporal dimensions can be achieved with Poisson-disk or random sampling. Both sampling schemes show similar aliasing patterns in the water/fat images. The maximum aliasing amplitude and the mean aliasing energy are 0.114 and 0.0018 for the Poisson-disk sampling, and 0.121 and 0.0026 for random sampling, respectively. Poisson disk sampling shows better uniformity and lower aliasing. b) The aliasing pattern for a single image with Poisson disk sampling with the same undersampling factor (the sampling pattern for the first echo of the sampling shown in a) is used here) shows higher aliasing. The maximum aliasing amplitude and mean aliasing energy are 0.197 and 0.0066, respectively.

reconstruction CS is performed on each individual echo image and the sampling pattern can be characterized by the corresponding PSF for a single echo $\hat{\mathbf{s}}_i = \mathbf{F}_u^H(1/\mathbf{\Theta})\mathbf{F}_u\mathbf{s}_i$. Fig. 6.2 b) shows the aliasing pattern in the first echo for the Poisson disk sampling pattern used in a). The aliasing in the echo images is significantly higher (factor 1.7 in the amplitude) compared to the aliasing in the water and fat images. An intuitive explanation for the decreased aliasing in the water and fat images is that combining the three echo images with different undersampling has an averaging effect, similar to noise averaging, so incoherent aliasing cancels out in the combined images. The reduced aliasing in the water and fat images suggests that the integrated CS-WF reconstruction is advantageous compared to a sequential reconstruction. If the same undersampling pattern is applied for all echoes, noise averaging still appears in the water and fat images, but the aliasing adds up coherently and is not reduced.

One potential sampling scheme for a 3D measurement with undersampling in $k_y - k_z - \text{TE}$ is schematically shown in Fig. 6.3.

A randomized multi-echo acquisition can be performed in a similar way as described in [110]. For example, the multi-gradient echo sequence shown in Fig. 6.3 could easily be modified by adding gradient blips (see zoomed area in Fig. 6.3) to shift the successive readouts in the phase encoding directions. Other schemes for 3D undersampling, like multi-echo acquisition with flyback gradients or single echo per TR are also conceivable.

6.3.3   Reconstruction

To jointly reconstruct the water and fat images and the field map from the undersampled data, the method proposed here applies a regularized nonlinear inversion. The combined CS-WF reconstruction problem can formally be defined as:

$$\underset{\mathbf{x}=[\boldsymbol{\rho}_w,\boldsymbol{\rho}_f,\boldsymbol{\phi}]}{\operatorname{argmin}} \{||g(\mathbf{x}) - \mathbf{y}||_2^2 + \lambda_w||\mathbf{\Psi}_w\boldsymbol{\rho}_w||_1 + \lambda_f||\mathbf{\Psi}_f\boldsymbol{\rho}_f||_1 + \lambda_\phi||\mathbf{\Phi}\boldsymbol{\phi}||_2^2\} \tag{6.15}$$

The first term accounts for data fidelity, where $g(\mathbf{x})$ is the nonlinear operator mapping the water and fat images and field map to the measured k-space data. Minimizing this term delivers the least squares solution, equivalent to the IDEAL reconstruction. The following two terms apply sparsity constraints on the water and fat images, which is the CS part of the reconstruction. The last term is a smoothness constraint applied on the field map. Different sparsifying transforms $\mathbf{\Psi}_w$ and $\mathbf{\Psi}_f$ can be applied on the water and fat images (e.g. wavelets for water and finite differences for fat) to account for the different structure in the images. In some cases, fat images are already sparse in the image domain and no additional transforms need to be applied (e.g. in the brain). Variations in the regularization parameters λ_w and λ_f could be used to improve the reconstruction for a given application. For instance, if the fat image is much sparser than the water image, a larger λ_f could be chosen. For simplicity, the general case is considered here, in which such prior information is not available and the same

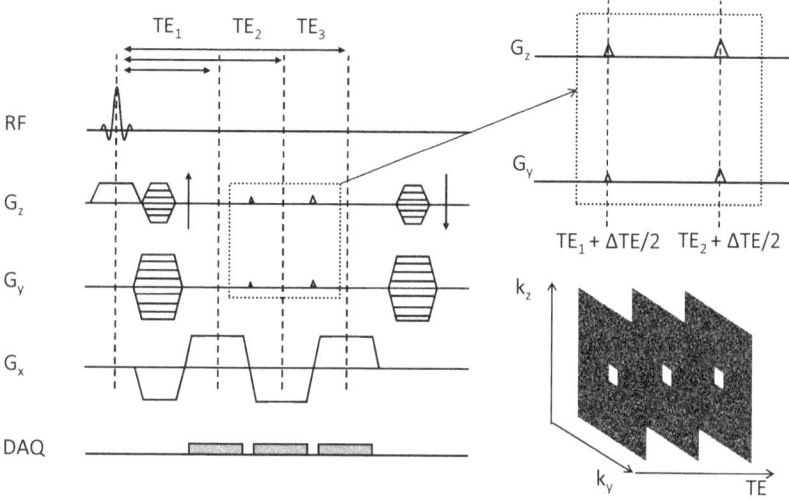

Figure 6.3. Schematic pulse sequence for three-point 3D water-fat chemical shift encoding using bipolar gradients for efficient data acquisition. Additional blips can be applied in G_y and G_z (see zoomed area) to achieve a random undersampling in the 3D $ky - kz -$ TE space.

sparsifying transform and regularization parameter for the water and fat images ($\boldsymbol{\Psi}_w = \boldsymbol{\Psi}_f$ and $\lambda_w = \lambda_f$) are applied. The second and third term can be combined as $\lambda_\rho || \boldsymbol{\Psi}\boldsymbol{\rho} ||_1$, where $\boldsymbol{\rho}$ contains both the water and fat images.

The proposed reconstruction approach applied to solve the problem in Eq. (6.15) iteratively approximates the nonlinear operator $g(\mathbf{x})$ with its linearized version, in a similar way as in the Gauss-Newton algorithm. At every iteration $g(\mathbf{x})$ is linearized around the current estimate $\mathbf{x}_n$

$$g(\mathbf{x}_n + d\mathbf{x}) \approx g(\mathbf{x}_n) + dg(\mathbf{x}_n)d\mathbf{x}, \tag{6.16}$$

where $dg(\mathbf{x}_n)$ is the Jacobian of $g(\mathbf{x})$ at the point $\mathbf{x}_n$. The modified problem

$$\operatorname*{argmin}_{d\mathbf{x}=[d\boldsymbol{\rho}_w, d\boldsymbol{\rho}_f, d\boldsymbol{\phi}]} \{ ||g(\mathbf{x}_n) + dg(\mathbf{x}_n)d\mathbf{x} - y||_2^2 + \lambda_\rho ||\boldsymbol{\Psi}(\boldsymbol{\rho}_n + d\boldsymbol{\rho})||_1 + \lambda_\phi ||\boldsymbol{\Phi}(\boldsymbol{\phi}_n + d\boldsymbol{\phi})||_2^2 \} \tag{6.17}$$

is then solved for the update $d\mathbf{x}$. A nonlinear conjugate gradient algorithm is used to solve Eq. (6.17). In the classical Gauss-Newton algorithm, the update is given by $\mathbf{x}_{n+1} = \mathbf{x}_n + d\mathbf{x}$. The update $d\mathbf{x}$ is a descent direction, but could be too large, resulting in a non-monotonic convergence of the algorithm. To assure monotonic convergence, the update $\mathbf{x}_{n+1} = \mathbf{x}_n + t d\mathbf{x}$ is used, where the step size t is determined by a backtracking line search.

The initialization of the algorithm has a twofold purpose. First, the problem is nonlinear and non-convex, so in the general case it is not guaranteed that a gradient-based method will lead to the correct solution. Second, starting with a good initial guess for the field map, the problem becomes "almost linear", and just a few iterations are sufficient to obtain a good solution. This is because the water-fat separation problem is linear when the field map is known.

A low-resolution initialization can be obtained by computing low resolution echo images from the fully sampled central part of k-space, performing conventional water-fat separation on these data, and interpolating the resulting images to the full resolution. Such low resolution initialization is usually good enough to lead to the correct solution. However, a large number of iterations may be necessary for the reconstruction. A high-resolution estimation can be obtained by using the decoupled reconstruction (performing CS in each individual echo image, followed by a conventional water-fat separation reconstruction) discussed above. This reconstruction shows some errors for larger reduction factors, but gives a good initialization of the CS-WF reconstruction greatly reducing the number of iterations.

In both cases, a reliable initial field map estimation is desirable. Possible values for the field map are obtained by an analytical determination of the minima of the voxel-wise cost function given in Eq. (6.6) through the roots of the polynomial $G(\phi(r)) = 0$, as described in the previous section. This results in two candidate maps for one period. Depending on the range of expected field variations one or several periods are considered.

The field map estimate is obtained by choosing values from the candidate maps under a local smoothness constraint. A region growing algorithm, similar to the one described in [161] is applied in this work. After obtaining the field map, the estimation of $\boldsymbol{\rho}$ is obtained by solving Eq. (6.1).

The data consistency of the reconstruction can be improved by enforcing the k-space data at the sampling locations to be equal to the originally acquired data at these locations in the last iteration. This way, the CS reconstruction is effectively used only to recover the missing data and is not allowed to modify the acquired data. Enforcing consistency with the measured data can recover some small coefficients that might be lost in the reconstruction and also recovers some of the noise of the original data. Since CS reconstruction also performs signal denoising, recovering some of the noise is often also perceived as visual improvement.

The CS-WF reconstruction is summarized below:

1. Initial field map estimation

    (a) extract low-resolution image or perform CS reconstruction for each echo

(b) compute possible field map values for each pixel and estimate initial field map using region growing

(c) estimate initial water and fat images using the results of (a) and (b)

2. Iteratively and simultaneously update the water and fat images and the field map, using the update given in Eq. (6.17)

3. Given the final estimate $\mathbf{x}_n$, compute a projection on k-space $\mathbf{y}_n = g(\mathbf{x}_n)$, set the measured data at the sampling locations $\mathbf{y}_n = \mathbf{y}|_{acq}$ and perform one last iteration.

6.4 Experiments

The proposed algorithm was implemented in C using the FFTW3 library. A second-order finite differences transform was used as a smoothness constraint on the field map. First-order finite differences (TV) were used as a sparsifying transform for the water and fat images. The raw data were normalized in the beginning of the reconstruction to make the choice of the regularization parameters insensitive to the data scaling. The empirically determined regularization parameters $\lambda_\rho = 0.02$ and $\lambda_\phi = 10^{-4}$ were used in the reconstruction. To reduce computation time and the effect of the noisy regions on the regularization parameters, the initial field map was computed only in regions with a signal amplitude above a certain threshold, determined by the estimated noise level (e.g. 1%). In the single-peak model the chemical shift of fat relative to water was assumed to be -220 Hz. For the multi-peak reconstruction, a three-peak model for fat was used. Frequencies of $(-30\text{Hz}, -165\text{Hz}, -210\text{Hz})$ with relative amplitudes $(0.15, 0.10, 0.75)$ at 1.5 T were used in the model as suggested by Brodsky et al. [165].

In vivo knee and abdominal data were acquired in healthy volunteers with their informed consent on a 1.5 T clinical scanner.

A 2D multi-slice turbo spin echo (TSE) sequence was used to image the knee with the following parameters: TR = 500 ms, TE = 21 ms, FOV= 160×160 mm^2, matrix size 256×256, 16 slices, slice thickness 3 mm, voxel size $0.6 \times 0.6 \times 3$ mm^3. Images were acquired at echo times of -0.4, 1.1, and 2.6 ms relative to the spin echo.

3D multi-gradient echo measurements were performed in the abdomen with the following parameters: $\text{TE}_1 = 1.8$ ms, Δ TE = 1.66 ms, TR = 6.9 ms, $\alpha = 15°$, FOV = $400 \times 320 \times 216$ mm^3, $240 \times 192 \times 54$ matrix, voxel size $1.6 \times 1.6 \times 4$ mm^3, sampling bandwidth 833 Hz/pixel. Before the data were passed to the reconstruction, inconsistencies between the odd and the even echoes were corrected using reference data measured just before the scan [154]. Using bipolar gradients, the chemical shift in even and odd echoes appears in opposite directions along the readout. However, with the acquisition bandwidth chosen for these measurements, this shift is in the sub-pixel range (0.26 pixels) and can be neglected. For larger shifts correction in k-space as suggested in [165] can be applied.

The data were retrospectively undersampled with several different reduction factors using Poisson disk sampling. Water-fat separation was performed using the CS-WF reconstruction for each reduction factor. In the case of full sampling, the sparsity transform regularization parameter was set to zero.

6.5 Results

The water and fat images and the field maps of the knee, obtained with CS-WF reconstruction at different reduction factors, are shown in Fig. 6.4. Uniform water-fat separation without any water-fat swaps was obtained at all reduction factors. High quality images could be obtained with up to a reduction factor of 2 in this two-dimensional case. A residual fat signal is seen in the water image due to the incomplete water-fat separation using the single-peak model.

Figure 6.5 shows the water images obtained with sequential reconstruction and CS-WF reconstruction for a reduction factor of two. The sequential reconstruction shows some residual artifacts in the low signal regions, whereas the CS-WF reconstruction results in an improved image quality. Note that the difference image for CS-WF (Fig. 6.5d) contains mostly noise, which could be explained with the denoising effect of CS reconstruction.

Fat appears very bright in TSE imaging [166], and the incomplete separation using a single-peak fat model leads to a decreased contrast in the water image. Reconstruction with a multi-peak fat model for an acceleration factor of 2 is shown in Fig. 6.6. The residual fat signal in the water image is significantly decreased, and the field map shows improved homogeneity (the jump at the water-fat interfaces is decreased).

Figure 6.7 shows the separated water and fat images for sample transversal and coronal slices of the 3D abdominal data. Images for full sampling and a reduction factor of 3 are shown, as well as difference images. An excellent image quality with uniform water-fat separation was obtained for the complete 3D dataset. The field map is shown for the coronal slice, which shows the highest field variations (feet-head gradient). The difference images show that the difference to the fully sampled image is small at relatively homogeneous regions with small variations of the water/fat content and is higher at the boundary regions. One reason for this is the smoothness constraint applied on the field map, which modifies the field map especially in these regions where discontinuities may occur. Another reason is that the ℓ_1 minimization penalizes large coefficients more than small ones causing larger errors in regions with large intensity variations, compared to more homogeneous ones.

Figure 6.8 shows the water images for another transversal slice of the abdominal 3D dataset, obtained with the CS-WF method for reduction factors of 3, 4 and 5. With increasing reduction factor, low contrast features gradually disappear (arrows). The loss of local contrast with increasing reduction factor is a known artifact of CS, caused by the loss of small coefficients in the transform domain, also reported in other works on CS [69]. With a low-resolution initialization, about 50 Gauss-Newton iterations are usually required. In the reconstruction

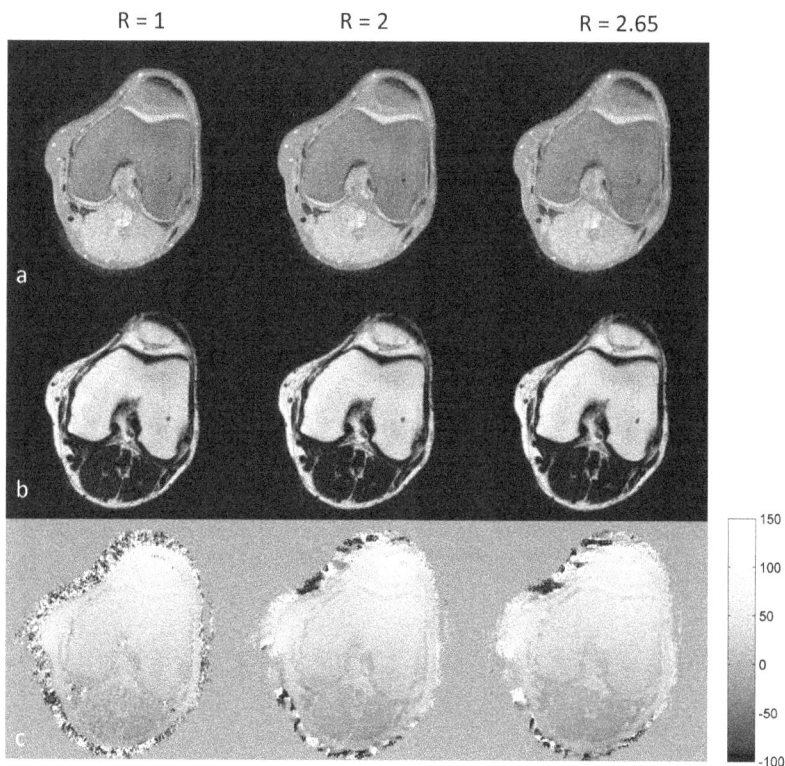

Figure 6.4. Water-fat separation with CS-WF in 2D knee data. **(a)** Water images, **(b)** fat images and **(c)** field maps reconstructed with CS-WF with reduction factors of 1, 2, and 2.65. The scale for the field map is given in Hz.

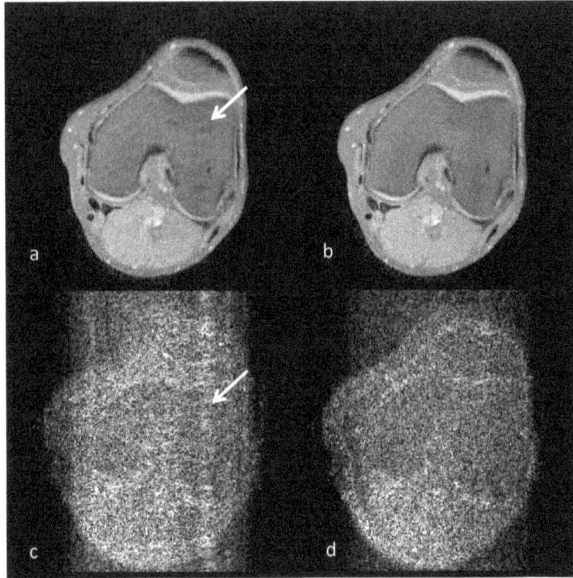

Figure 6.5. 2D CS water-fat separation with R = 2. The water image obtained with sequential reconstruction (CS on each echo, followed by water-fat separation) shows some residual artifacts, which are visible in the bone marrow (**a**). The image obtained with the integrated CS-WF reconstruction has an improved image quality (**b**). Difference images (amplified by a factor of 10) with respect to the fully sampled water image are shown in (**c**) and (**d**).

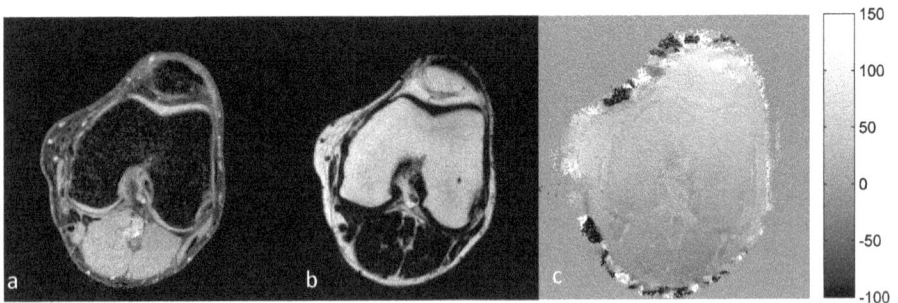

Figure 6.6. 2D CS-WF reconstruction with R = 2 and multi-peak fat modeling. Multi-peak fat modeling results in a significant improvement of the water-fat separation, especially in the case of high intensity fat signal, as typical e.g. in TSE imaging.

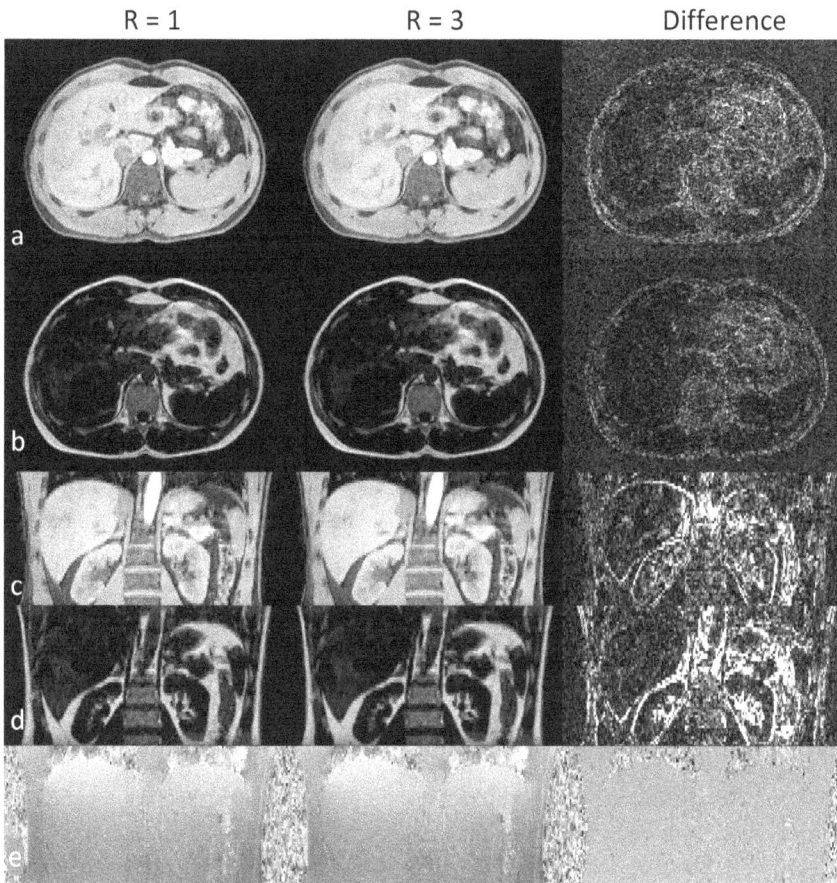

Figure 6.7. CS-WF reconstruction of 3D abdominal data with R = 3. Separated water and fat images with full sampling and a reduction factor of 3 are shown for a transversal (**a,b**) and a coronal slice (**c,d**) from a 3D abdominal dataset. The field map for the coronal slice is shown in (**e**). Difference images are amplified by a factor of 10 for better visualization.

of the images presented above, high-resolution initialization was used, reducing the number of iterations to 5. With the current implementation, the computation time for one Gauss-Newton step for the 3D data is 9 min (CPU 2.4 GHz, 16 GByte RAM).

R = 3   R = 4   R = 5

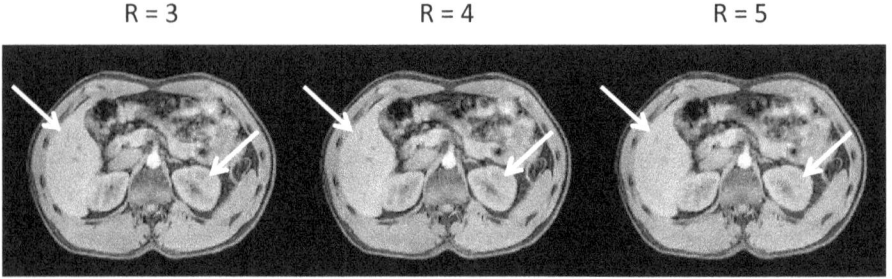

Figure 6.8. CS-WF reconstruction of 3D abdominal data with different reduction factors. Water images obtained with CS-WF for reduction factors of 3, 4 and 5 are shown. Increasing the reduction factor results in loss of contrast (arrows) and eventually residual aliasing artifacts.

6.6   Discussion

In this chapter, a method for water-fat decomposition from undersampled data was presented, which simultaneously recovers the missing k-space data and performs a water-fat separation. The method was demonstrated on in vivo 2D turbo spin echo knee data and 3D multi-gradient echo abdominal data. A reduction factor of 3 can be achieved for 3D measurements facilitating water-fat separation with three-point measurements in a total scan time that could be comparable or even less than the time for acquiring a single 3D image.

The reduced aliasing with randomized sampling in the chemical shift encoding direction and better sparsity in the water and fat images allow an improved performance of CS if these are exploited in the reconstruction. This improvement of the CS-WF reconstruction over sequentially applying CS and the water-fat separation, gained by exploiting the chemical shift encoding dimension in the reconstruction, has been demonstrated on in vivo data.

An efficient multi-gradient-echo scheme with bipolar gradients was considered in this work, which allows short TR and inter-echo spacing. While this sampling is highly efficient and allows a short scan time, some issues such as trajectory misalignment due to gradient delays and opposite chemical shift artifacts in the even/odd echoes might arise, and appropriate corrections for differences in the k-space trajectories in the even/odd echoes [154, 155] and compensation for the chemical shift artifacts in k-space [165, 167] should be applied, where necessary. Other sampling schemes like multi-echo sampling with flyback gradients or single echo sampling can avoid some of the previously mentioned problems at the cost of longer scan time.

An extension to parallel imaging could further improve the imaging speed. Several works have proposed a combined CS parallel imaging reconstruction by either incorporating the sensitivity encoding matrix in the reconstruction or by using auto-calibration methods [93, 94]. The different principles of parallel imaging and CS cause different problems at high accelerations. The acceleration in parallel imaging is mainly limited by SNR. CS reduces noise, but at high accelerations starts to lose small coefficients. A combined CS-PI reconstruction allows higher acceleration than each of the methods alone [93, 94]. Therefore, a fully integrated CS-PI-WF reconstruction is expected to provide the highest acceleration for this problem. A combination with parallel imaging for 3D reconstruction might be challenging in terms of memory requirements and computation speed, especially for large number of coil elements. Applying parallel computing using multiprocessors or dedicated hardware systems could be helpful to address this problem. These investigations are subject of future work.

Reliable water-fat separation is a difficult problem because of the inherent ambiguity in the field map estimation, and the CS-WF reconstruction must also deal with these difficulties. A field map estimation, obtained by explicitly locating the possible field map values has been shown to yield a more robust solution than descent based methods [161–163]. We have shown that such an approach provides a good initialization for the CS-WF reconstruction, avoiding swaps of water and fat in the separation. Furthermore, field map smoothness and data consistency are utilized during the CS-WF reconstruction.

An extension to a multi-peak fat model shows improved water-fat separation as expected. The multi-peak fat model also improves the data consistency, which is advantageous for the stability of the reconstruction. In this case, the water and fat images are almost complementary, which might potentially be used to formulate an additional constraint in the reconstruction. For anatomies in which the fat image is very sparse (e.g. brain), it might be useful to apply a sparsity constraint directly in the image domain. However, for large reduction factors this constraint might bias very small fat fractions toward zero.

The CS-WF method was demonstrated for three-point measurements acquiring complex water and fat images and a field map. The method is generally applicable for different number of echoes. For two-point measurements, the additional chemical shift encoding direction is reduced to only two echoes. Therefore, it is expected that the advantage of a joint reconstruction as proposed here over a sequential reconstruction will be reduced. Another possible difficulty is that the signal model in two-point water-fat separation methods is less accurate, which could reduce the performance of the reconstruction. Increasing the number of echoes might improve the data consistency by incorporating a more complex data model, e.g. a multi-peak fat model, in which the amplitudes at different resonance frequencies are estimated in the reconstruction. For a higher number of echoes, one could also consider a spectroscopic approach, which is linear and would allow using a different type of reconstruction like the one presented in [168]. Such spectroscopic approaches will generally require more measurements, but might be more robust in terms of field map estimation.

CHAPTER SEVEN

SUMMARY AND OUTLOOK

It is typical of the unintelligent man to insist on assembling complete sets of everything. Imperfect sets are better. In everything, no matter what it may be, uniformity is undesirable. Leaving something incomplete makes it interesting and gives one the feeling that there is room for growth.

— KEIKO, ESSAYS IN IDLENESS, 14TH CENTURY

7.1 Summary

Recent advances in sampling theory, known as compressed sensing, have shown a great potential to exploit the inherent redundancy of signals to improve sampling efficiency. The ability to acquire reduced amount of data without significantly decreasing image quality is of significant importance in MRI since imaging time is a critical factor in many MRI applications.

A generalized approach for the application of CS in MRI, which focuses on the acquisition of a single image using a general purpose sparsifying transform usually provides only a limited sampling acceleration. The pursuit for maximum acceleration, measuring as few data as possible, requires optimization of the data acquisition and the applied sparsifying transform to the specific application. The wide variety of MR applications, presenting different types of contrast and structures in the images, as well as additional sampling dimensions, such as temporal, parametric, or spectral dimensions, require the development of methods that efficiently exploit the data redundancy and the higher dimensional sampling.

This work presented new methods for the application of CS in MRI, which allow to better exploit the potential of CS to improve imaging speed of MRI.

Radial sampling with golden ratio profile ordering was suggested as a practical trajectory for CS that allows undersampling in all spatial dimensions. Golden ratio radial sampling achieves more incoherent aliasing than uniform radial sampling. Furthermore, it provides a nearly uniform profile distribution for any arbitrary selection of data from a dynamic acquisition. This allows for retrospective adjustment of the temporal resolution and position of reconstruction time frames according to the actual temporal dynamics of the signal, without the need for prior planning. CS in combination with parallel imaging and golden ratio sampling has shown potential for improving the temporal resolution in dynamic imaging.

Training a sparsifying transform for a specific application results in better sparsity and therefore higher achievable acceleration factors in CS. A method for training a model-based sparsifying transform in MR parameter mapping was presented, which allowed a significant reduction of the required data without compromising the quality of the parameter maps. The method was demonstrated for the example of in vivo relaxation parameter mapping. Further studies are needed to expand the scope of possible MR parameters (e.g. diffusion, perfusion) that can be addressed with this new concept.

A new reconstruction method for integrated CS and water-fat separation (CS-WF) was presented as an example for reconstruction based on nonlinear measurements. Its feasibility was demonstrated in three-point measurements performed in 2D and 3D in vivo applications. The CS-WF reconstruction offers a promising framework for scan time reduction in water-fat separation applications that are not SNR critical. This can be interesting for a couple of clinical applications.

7.2 Outlook

This work demonstrated the feasibility of the proposed methods in simulations and in experiments with volunteers. Further research is necessary before these approaches can be adopted in clinical practice. An important step for the future development of the methods presented in this work, as well as CS-MRI in general, is the reduction of the reconstruction times. This goal can be pursued both in terms of faster algorithms and by using multi-processors and dedicated hardware.

The idea of adapting the acquisition and reconstruction to a specific application can be exploited in multiple ways. This could be achieved for instance by applying further prior knowledge in the reconstruction, e.g. in the form of initialization. Another option is tailoring the sampling density according to statistics over previously acquired training data. The prior knowledge used in the reconstruction should be specific to the application, but as general as possible, to avoid undesired errors in the image due to the reconstruction.

Furthermore, combination of CS with other methods for fast imaging, such as parallel imaging, is of great importance. Although methods for combined CS and PI reconstruction already exist, it is subject of future research to gain better understanding of how the additional encoding in parallel imaging combines with sparsity driven reconstruction.

Iterative reconstruction methods as the ones in CS-MRI rely on the consistency of the measured data with the measurement model. Therefore, the accuracy of the reconstruction depends on the knowledge of the sampling trajectory. Applying an accurate information about the actual sampling trajectory is especially important in non-Cartesian imaging and improvements in this field could be very advantageous for the application of non-Cartesian trajectories in CS.

An important step toward the clinical applicability of CS-MRI is identifying clinical applications that could benefit from CS and validating the methods on clinical data.

It is difficult to predict the future of CS and its applications in MRI. This very young theory has gained the attention of many researchers and we are witnessing an amazing development of both theory and applications in parallel. What is clear is that CS has awaken a new interest in irregular sampling patterns, in iterative reconstruction methods, and in methods applying prior knowledge in the reconstruction. The ability of these methods to improve image quality and their potential for faster imaging are expected to be highly valuable in improving diagnostic imaging.

Bibliography

[1] D. Twieg, "The k-trajectory formulation of the NMR imaging process with applications in analysis and synthesis of imaging methods", *Med Phys*, vol. 10, pp. 610–621, 1983.

[2] S. Ljunggren, "A simple graphical representation of Fourier-based imaging methods", *J Magn Reson*, vol. 54, pp. 338–343, 1983.

[3] J. Pauly, D. Nishimura, A. Macovski, "A k-space analysis of small-tip-angle excitations", *J Magn Reson*, vol. 81, pp. 43–56, 1989.

[4] P. Lauterbur, "Image Formation by induced local interactions: Examples employing nuclear magnetic resonance", *Nature*, vol. 242, pp. 190–191, 1973.

[5] G. Glover & J. Pauly, "Projection reconstruction techniques for reduction of motion effects in MRI", *Magn Reson Med*, vol. 28, pp. 275–289, 1992.

[6] C. Ahn, J. Kim, Z. Cho, "High-speed spiral-scan echo planar NMR imaging", *IEEE Trans Med Imaging*, vol. 5, pp. 2–7, 1986.

[7] C. Meyer, B. Hu, D. Nishimura, A. Macovski, "Fast spiral coronary artery imaging", *Magn Reson Med*, vol. 28, pp. 202–213, 1992.

[8] C. Tsai & D. Nishimura, "Reduced aliasing artifacts using variable-density k-space sampling trajectories", *Magn Reson Med*, vol. 43, pp. 452–458, 2000.

[9] J. Pipe, "Motion correction with PROPELLER MRI: application to head motion and free breathing cardiac imaging", *Magn Reson Med*, vol. 42, pp. 963–969, 1999.

[10] D. Noll, D. Nishimura, A. Mackovski, "Homodyne detection in magnetic resonance imaging", *IEEE Trans Med Imaging*, vol. 10, pp. 154–164, 1991.

[11] R. Likes, "Moving gradient zeugmatography", US Patent 4307343, 1981.

[12] K. Scheffler & J. Hennig, "Frequency resolved single-shot MR imaging using stochastic k-space trajectories", *Magn Reson Med*, vol. 35, pp. 569–576, 1996.

[13] A. Papoulis, "Generalized sampling expansion", *IEEE Trans Circ Syst*, vol. 24, pp. 652–654, 1977.

[14] A. Barger, W. Block, Y. Toporov, T. Grist, C. Mistretta, "Time-resolved contrast-enhanced imaging with isotropic resolution and broad coverage using an undersampled 3D projection trajectory", *Magn Reson Med*, vol. 48, pp. 297–305, 2002.

[15] J. O'Sullivan, "A fast sinc function gridding algorithm for Fourier inversion in computer tomography", *IEEE Trans Med Imag*, vol. 4, pp. 200–207, 1985.

[16] J. Jackson, C. Meyer, Nishimura D., Machowski A., "Selection of a convolution function for Fourier inversion using gridding", *IEEE Trans Med Imaging*, vol. 10, pp. 473–478, 1991.

[17] P. Roemer, W. Edelstein, C. Hayes, S. Souza, O. Mueller, "The NMR phased array", *Magn Reson Med*, vol. 16, pp. 192–225, 1990.

[18] B. Chronik & B. Rutt, "Simple linear formulation for magnetostimulation specific to MRI gradient coils", *Magn Reson Med*, vol. 45, pp. 916–919, 2001.

[19] P. Mansfield, "Multi-planar image-formation using NMR spin echoes", *J Phys C:Solid state phys*, vol. 10, pp. L55–L58, 1977.

[20] D. Sodickson & W. Manning, "Simultaneous acquisition of spatial harmonics (SMASH): Fast imaging with radiofrequency coil arrays", *Magn Reson Med*, vol. 38, pp. 591–603, 1997.

[21] K. Pruessmann, M. Weiger, M. Scheidegger, P. Boesiger, "SENSE: Sensitivity encoding for fast MRI", *Magn Reson Med*, vol. 42, pp. 952–962, 1999.

[22] M. Griswold, P. Jakob, R. Heidemann, M. Nittka, V. Jellus, J. Wang, B. Kiefer, A. Haase, "Generalized autocalibrating partially parallel acquisitions (GRAPPA)", *Magn Reson Med*, vol. 47, pp. 1202–1210, 2002.

[23] M. Schmitt, A. Potthast, D. Sosnovik, J. Polimeni, G. Wiggins, C. Triantafyllou, L. Wald, "A 128-channel receive-only cardiac coil for highly accelerated cardiac MRI at 3 Tesla", *Magn Reson Med*, vol. 59, pp. 1431–9, 2008.

[24] C. Hardy, R. Giaquinto, J. Piel, K. Rohling, L. Marinelli, D. Blezek, E. Fiveland, R. Darrow, T. Foo, "128-channel body MRI with a flexible high-density receiver-coil array", *J Magn Reson Imaging*, vol. 28, pp. 1431–9, 2008.

[25] D. Feinberg, J. Hale, J. Watts, L. Kaufman, A. Mark, "Halving MR imaging time by conjugation: demonstration at 3.5 kG", *Radiology*, vol. 161, pp. 527–531, 1986.

[26] J. Cuppen & A. van Est, "Reducing MR imaging time by one-sided reconstruction", *Magn Reson Imaging*, vol. 5, pp. 526–527, 1987.

[27] J. van Vaals, M. Brummer, W. Dixon, H. Tuithof, H. Engels, R. Nelson, B. Gerety, J. Chezmar, J. den Boer, "Keyhole method for accelerating imaging of contrast agent uptake", *J Magn Reson Imaging*, vol. 3, pp. 671–675, 1993.

[28] R. Jones, O. Haraldseth, T. Müller, P. Rinck, A. Oksendal, "K-space substitution: a novel dynamic imaging technique.", *Magn Reson Med*, vol. 29, pp. 830–834., 1993.

[29] Z.P. Liang & P. Lauterbur, "An efficient method for dynamic magnetic resonance imaging", *IEEE Trans Med Imaging*, vol. 13, pp. 677–686, 1994.

[30] J. Tsao, P. Boesiger, K. Pruessmann, "k-t BLAST and k-t SENSE: dynamic MRI with high frame rate exploiting spatiotemporal correlations", *Magn Reson Med*, vol. 50, pp. 1021–1042, 2003.

[31] H. Pedersen, S. Kozerke, S. Ringgaard, K. Nehrke, W. Kim, "k-t PCA: temporally constrained k-t BLAST reconstruction using principal component analysis", *Magn Reson Med*, vol. 62, pp. 706–716, 2009.

[32] C. Mistretta, O. Wieben, J. Velikina, W. Block, J. Perry, Y. Wu, "Highly constrained backprojection for time-resolved MRI", *Magn Reson Med*, vol. 55, pp. 30–40, 2006.

[33] E. Candés & T. Tao, "Near-optimal signal recovery from random projections: universal encoding strategies?", *IEEE Trans Inf Theory*, vol. 52, pp. 5406–5425, 2006.

[34] D. Donoho, "Compressed sensing", *IEEE Trans Inf Theory*, vol. 52, pp. 1289–1306, 2006.

[35] C. Shannon, "Communication in the presence of noise", pp. 10–21, 1949.

[36] H. Landau, "Necessary density conditions for sampling and interpolation of certain entire functions", *Acta Math*, vol. 117, pp. 37–52, 1967.

[37] P. Feng & Y. Bresler, "Spectrum-blind minimum-rate sampling and reconstruction of multiband signals", in *Proc IEEE Int Conf ASSP*, vol. 3, Atlanta, GA , USA, pp. 1688–1691, 1996.

[38] Y. Bresler & P. Feng, "Spectrum-blind minimum-rate sampling and reconstruction of 2-d multiband signals", in *Proc IEEE Int Conf on Image Proc*, vol. 1, Lausanne, Switzerland, pp. 701–704, 1996.

[39] R. Venkataramani & Y. Bresler, "Further results on spectrum blind sampling of 2d signals", in *Proc IEEE Int Conf on Image Proc*, vol. 2, Chicago, IL, USA, pp. 752–756, 1998.

[40] G. Wallace, "The JPEG still picture compression standard", *Communications of the ACM*, vol. 34, pp. 30–44, 1991.

[41] D. Taubman & M. Marcellin, *JPEG2000 : Image Compression Fundamentals, Standards and Practice.*, Kluwer Academic Publishers, Boston, 2002.

[42] Stéphane Mallat, *A Wavelet Tour of Signal Processing*, Academic Press, 1999.

[43] R. Baraniuk, M. Davenport, R. DeVore, M. Wakin, "A simple proof of the restricted isometry property for random matrices", *Constr Approx*, vol. 28, pp. 253–263, 2008.

[44] S. Mendelson, A. Pajor, N. Tomczak-Jaegermann, "Uniform uncertainty principle for Bernoulli and subgaussian ensembles", *Constr Approx*, vol. 28, pp. 277–289, 2008.

[45] M. Rudelson & R. Vershynin, "On sparse reconstruction from Fourier and Gaussian measurements", *Comm Pure Appl Math*, vol. 61, pp. 1025–1045, 2008.

[46] R. Coifman, F. Geshwind, Y. Meyer, "Noiselets", *Appl Comput Harmon Anal*, vol. 10, pp. 27–44, 2001.

[47] E. Candès & T. Tao, "Decoding by linear programming", *IEEE Trans Inf Theory*, vol. 51, pp. 4203–4215, 2005.

[48] D. Donoho & M. Elad, "Optimally sparse representation in general (non-orthogonal) dictionaries via ℓ_1 minimization", *Proc Natl Acad Sci*, vol. 100, pp. 2197–2202, 2002.

[49] E. Candés, Y. Eldar, D. Needell, "Compressed Sensing with Coherent and Redundant Dictionaries", *Submitted for publication*, 2010.

[50] M. Elad, P. Milanfar, R. Rubinstein, "Analysis versus synthesis in signal priors", in *Inverse Problems*, vol. 23, pp. 947–968, 2007.

[51] E. Candés, M. Wakin, S. Boyd, "Enhancing sparsity by reweighted ℓ_1 minimization", *J of Fourier Anal and App (Special issue on sparsity)*, vol. 14, pp. 877–905, 2008.

[52] G. Davis, S. Mallat, M. Avellaneda, "Adaptive greedy approximations", *Constr Approx*, vol. 13, pp. 57–98, 1997.

[53] S. Chen, D. Donoho, M. Saunders, "Atomic Decomposition by basis pursuit", *SIAM J Sci Comput*, vol. 20, pp. 33–61, 1999.

[54] E. Candés, J. Romberg, T. Tao, "Robust uncertainty principles:Exact signal recovery from highly incomplete frequency information", *IEEE Trans Inf Theory*, vol. 52, pp. 489–509, 2006.

[55] S. Mallat & Z. Zhang, "Matching pursuit with time-frequency dictionaries", *IEEE Trans Signal Process*, vol. 41, pp. 3397–3415, 1993.

[56] J. Tropp, "Greed is Good: Algorithmic results for sparse approximation", *IEEE Trans on Inf Theory*, vol. 50, pp. 2231–2242, 2004.

[57] R. Chartrand, "Exact reconstruction of sparse signals via nonconvex minimization", *IEEE Signal Process Lett*, vol. 14, pp. 707–710, 2007.

[58] I. Daubechies, M. Defrise, C. De Mol, "An iterative thresholding algorithm for linear inverse problems with a sparsity constraint", *Comm Pure Appl Math*, vol. 57, pp. 1413–1457, 2004.

[59] C. Lawson, *Contributions to the theory of linear least maximum approximations*, Ph.D. thesis, UCLA, 1961.

[60] A. Beaton & J. Tukey, "The fitting of power series, meaning polynomials, illustrated on bandspectroscopic data", *Technometrics*, vol. 16, pp. 147–185, 1974.

[61] B. Rao & K. Kreutz-Delgado, "An affine scaling methodology for best basis selection", *IEEE Trans Signal Processing*, vol. 47, pp. 187–200, 1999.

[62] I. Daubechies, R. DeVore, M. Fornasier, S. Gunturk, "Iteratively re-weighted least squares minimization for sparse recovery", *Comm Pure Appl Math*, vol. 63, pp. 1–38, 2010.

[63] M. Elad, "Why simple shrinkage is still relevant for redundant representations", *IEEE Trans Inf Theory*, vol. 52, pp. 5559–5569, 2006.

[64] M. Elad, B. Matalon, M. Zibulevsky, "Coordinate and subspace optimization methods for linear least squares with non-quadratic regularization", *Appl Comput Harmon Anal*, vol. 23, pp. 346–367, 2007.

[65] M. Figueiredo & R. Nowak, "An em algorithm for wavelet-based image restoration", *IEEE Trans Image Processing*, vol. 12, pp. 906–916, 2003.

[66] M. Figueiredo & R. Nowak, "A bound optimization approach to wavelet-based image deconvolution", *IEEE International Conference on Image Processing*, pp. 782–785, 2006.

[67] D. Donoho, "For most large underdetermined systems of equations, the minimal ℓ_1-norm near-solution approximates the sparsest near-solution", *Comm Pure Appl Math*, vol. 907, p. 934, 2006.

[68] S. Boyd & L. Vandenberghe, *Convex Optimization*, Cambridge University Press, Boston, 2004.

[69] M. Lustig, D. Donoho, J. Pauly, "Sparse MRI: The application of compressed sensing for rapid MR imaging", *Magn Reson Med*, vol. 58, pp. 1182–95, 2007.

[70] E. Candés & J. Romberg, "Practical signal recovery from random projections", in *Proceedings of the SPIE Conference on Wavelet Applications in Signal and Image Processing XI*, San Diego, CA, USA, 2004.

[71] M. Osborne, B. Presnell, B. Turlach, "On the LASSO and its dual", *J Comput Graph Statist*, vol. 9, pp. 319–337, 2000.

[72] K. Koh, S. Kim, S. Boyd, "Solver for ℓ_1-regularized least squares problems", Tech. Rep., Stanford University, 2007.

[73] E. Candés, "ℓ_1-magic", Tech. Rep., Caltech, 2007.

[74] J. Tropp & A. Gilbert, "Signal Recovery From Random Measurements Via Orthogonal Matching Pursuit", *IEEE Trans Inf Theory*, vol. 53, pp. 4655–4666, 2007.

[75] D. Donoho, Y. Tsaig, I. Drori, J. Starck, "Sparse solution of underdetermined linear equations by stagewise Orthogonal Matching Pursuit (StOMP)", Tech. Rep., Departement of Statistics Stanford University, 2006.

[76] D. Needell & R. Vershynin, "Uniform uncertainty principle and signal recovery via regularized orthogonal matching pursuit", *Found of Comp Mathematics*, vol. 9, pp. 317–334, 2009.

[77] D. Needell & J. Tropp, "CoSaMP: Iterative signal recovery from incomplete and inaccurate samples", *Appl Comput Harmon Anal*, vol. 26, pp. 1–30, 2008.

[78] Y. Pati, R. Rezaiifar, P. Krishnaprasad, "Orthogonal Matching Pursuit: Recursive function approximation with applications to wavelet decomposition", in *Proceeding of the 27th Annual Asilomar Conference on Signals, Systems and Computers*, pp. 40–44, 1993.

[79] I. Gorodnitsky & B. Rao, "Sparse signal reconstruction from limited data using FOCUSS: A re-weighted norm minimization algorithm", *IEEE Trans Signal Processing*, vol. 45, pp. 600–616, 1997.

[80] J. Trzasko & A. Manduca, "Highly undersampled magnetic resonance image reconstruction via homotopic L0-minimization", *IEEE Trans Med Imaging*, vol. 28, pp. 106–121, 2009.

[81] T. Blumensath & M. Davies, "Iterative hard thresholding for compressed sensing", *Appl Computat Harmon Anal*, vol. 27, pp. 265–274, 2009.

[82] M. Fornasier & H. Rauhut, "Iterative thresholding algorithms", *Appl Comput Harmon Anal*, vol. 25, pp. 187–208, 2008.

[83] M. Zibulevsky & M. Elad, "L1-L2 optimization in image and signal processing", *IEEE Signal Processing Magazine*, vol. 27, pp. 76–88, 2010.

[84] J. Haldar, D. Hernando, B. Sutton, Z.-P. Liang, "Data acquisition considerations for compressed sensing in MRI", in *Proceedings of the 16th Annual Meeting of ISMRM*, Berlin, Germany, 2007.

[85] F. Sebert, Y. Zou, B. Liu, L. Ying, "Compressed sensing MRI with random B1 field", in *Proceedings of the 16th Annual Meeting of ISMRM*, Toronto, Canada, 2008.

[86] D. Liang, G. Xu, H. Wang, K. King, D. Xu, L. Ying, "Toeplitz random encoding MR imaging using compressed sensing", in *Proceedings of the IEEE International Symposium on Biomedical Imaging*, Boston, MA, USA, 2009.

[87] F. Knoll, C. Clason, R. Stollberger, "Tailored 3D Random Sampling Patterns for Nonlinear Parallel Imaging", in *Proceedings of the 18th Annual Meeting of ISMRM*, Stockholm, Sweden, p. 2876, 2010.

[88] C. Zhao, T. Lang, J. Ji, "Compressed Sensing Parallel Imaging", in *Proceedings of the 16th Annual Meeting of ISMRM*, Toronto, Canada, p. 1478, 2008.

[89] B. Wu, R. Millane, R. Watts, P. Bones, "Applying Compressed Sensing in Parallel MRI", in *Proceedings of the 16th Annual Meeting of ISMRM*, Toronto, Canada, p. 1480, 2008.

[90] L. Marinelli, C. Hardy, D. Blezek, "MRI with Accelerated Multi-Coil Compressed Sensing", in *Proceedings of the 16th Annual Meeting of ISMRM*, Toronto, Canada, p. 1484, 2008.

[91] K. King, "Combining Compressed Sensing and Parallel Imaging", in *Proceedings of the 16th Annual Meeting of ISMRM*, Toronto, Canada, p. 1488, 2008.

[92] B. Liu, F. Sebert, Y. Zou, L. Ying, "SparseSENSE: Randomly-Sampled Parallel Imaging Using Compressed Sensing", in *Proceedings of the 16th Annual Meeting of ISMRM*, Toronto, Canada, p. 3154, 2008.

[93] D. Liang, B. Liu, J. Wang, L. Ying, "Accelerating SENSE using compressed sensing", *Magn Reson Med*, vol. 62, pp. 1574–1584, 2009.

[94] M. Lustig, M. Alley, S. Vasanawala, D. Donoho, J. Pauly, "L1 SPIR-IT: Autocalibrating Parallel Imaging Compressed Sensing", in *Proceedings of the 17th Annual Meeting of ISMRM*, Honolulu, Hawaii, p. 379, 2009.

[95] A. Fischer, N. Seiberlich, M. Blaimer, P. Jakob, F. Breuer, M. Griswold, "A Combination of Nonconvex Compressed Sensing and GRAPPA (CS-GRAPPA)", in *Proceedings of the 17th Annual Meeting of ISMRM*, Honolulu, Hawaii, p. 2813, 2009.

[96] M. Uecker, K. Block, J. Frahm, "Non-linear inversion with L1 wavelet regularization- Application to autocalibrated parallel imaging", in *Proceedings of the 16th Annual Meeting of ISMRM*, Toronto, Canada, p. 1479, 2008.

[97] J. Trzasko, C. Haider, E. Borisch, S. Riederer, A. Manduca, "Nonconvex Compressive Sensing with Parallel Imaging for Highly Accelerated 4D CE-MRA", in *Proceedings of the 18th Annual Meeting of ISMRM*, Stockholm, Sweden, p. 347, 2010.

[98] U. Gamper, P. Boesiger, S. Kozerke, "Compressed sensing in dynamic MRI", *Magn Reson Med*, vol. 59, pp. 365–373, 2008.

[99] H. Jung, K. Sung, K. Nayak, E. Kim, J. Ye, "k-t FOCUSS: A general compressed sensing framework for high resolution dynamic MRI", *Magn Reson Med*, vol. 61, pp. 103–116, 2009.

[100] P. Lai, M. Lustig, A. Brau, S. Vasanawala, "kt SPIRiT for Ultra-Fast Cardiac Cine Imaging with Prospective or Retrospective Cardiac Gating", in *Proceedings of the 18th Annual Meeting of ISMRM*, Stockholm, Sweden, p. 482, 2010.

[101] M. Doneva, J. Sénégas, P. Börnert, H. Eggers, A. Mertins, "Accelerated MR Parameter Mapping Using Compressed Sensing with Model-Based Sparsifying Transform", in *Proceedings of the 17th Annual Meeting of ISMRM*, Honolulu, Hawaii, p. 2812, 2009.

[102] C. Huang, C. Graff, A. Bilgin, M. Altbach, "Fast MR Parameter Mapping from Highly Undersampled Data by Direct Reconstruction of Principal Component Coefficient Maps Using Compressed Sensing", in *Proceedings of the 18th Annual Meeting of ISMRM*, Stockholm, Sweden, p. 348, 2010.

[103] J. Velikina, A. Alexander, A. Samsonov, "A Novel Approach for T1 Relaxometry Using Constrained Reconstruction in Parametric Dimension", in *Proceedings of the 18th Annual Meeting of ISMRM*, Stockholm, Sweden, p. 350, 2010.

[104] L. Feng, R. Otazo, J. Jensen, D. Sodickson, D. Kim, "Accelerated Breath-Hold Multi-Echo FSE Pulse Sequence Using Compressed Sensing and Parallel Imaging for T2 Measurement in the Heart", in *Proceedings of the 18th Annual Meeting of ISMRM*, Stockholm, Sweden, p. 351, 2010.

[105] M. Menzel, K. Khare, K. King, X. Tao, C. Hardy, L. Marinelli, "Accelerated Diffusion Spectrum Imaging in the Human Brain Using Compressed Sensing", in *Proceedings of the 18th Annual Meeting of ISMRM*, Stockholm, Sweden, p. 1698, 2010.

[106] B. Wilkins & M. Singh, "Diffusion Histogram as a Marker of Fiber Crossing Within a Voxel", in *Proceedings of the 18th Annual Meeting of ISMRM*, Stockholm, Sweden, p. 1699, 2010.

[107] K. King & W. Sun, "Compressed Sensing with Vascular Phase Contrast Acquisition", in *Proceedings of the 17th Annual Meeting of ISMRM*, Honolulu, Hawaii, p. 2817, 2009.

[108] K. Khare, C. Hardy, K. King, P. Turski, L. Marinelli, "Accelerated 3D Phase-Contrast Imaging Using Adaptive Compressed Sensing with No Free Parameters", in *Proceedings of the 18th Annual Meeting of ISMRM*, Stockholm, Sweden, p. 346, 2010.

[109] L. Marinelli, K. Khare, K. King, C. Hardy, "Breath-Held Highly-Accelerated 2D Fourier-Velocity Encoded MRI Using Compressed Sensing", in *Proceedings of the 18th Annual Meeting of ISMRM*, Stockholm, Sweden, p. 4872, 2010.

[110] S. Hu, M. Lustig, A. Chen, J. Crane, A. Kerr, D. Kelley, R. Hurd, J. Kurhanewitz, S. Nelson, J. Pauly, D. Vigneron, "Compressed sensing for resolution enhancement of hyperpolarized 13C flyback 3D-MRSI", *J Magn Reson*, vol. 192, pp. 258–264, 2008.

[111] S. Hu, M. Lustig, A. Balakrishnan, P. Larson, R. Bok, J. Kurhanewitz, S. Nelson, A. Goga, J. Pauly, D. Vigneron, "3D compressed sensing for highly accelerated hyperpolarized 13C MRSI with in vivo applications to transgenic mouse models of cancer", *Magn Reson Med*, vol. 63, pp. 312–321, 2008.

[112] S. Ajraoui, K. Lee, M. Deppe, S. Parnell, J. Rarra-Robles, J. Wild, "Compressed sensing in hyperpolarized 3He Lung MRI", *Magn Reson Med*, vol. 63, pp. 1059–1069, 2010.

[113] M. Doneva, P. Börnert, H. Eggers, A. Mertins, J. Pauly, M. Lustig, "CS-Dixon: Compressed Sensing for Water-Fat Dixon Reconstruction", in *Proceedings of the 18th Annual Meeting of ISMRM*, Stockholm, Sweden, p. 2919, 2010.

[114] S. Sharma, H. Hu, K. Nayak, "Acceleration of IDEAL Water-Fat Imaging Using Compressed Sensing", in *Proceedings of the 18th Annual Meeting of ISMRM*, Stockholm, Sweden, p. 4884, 2010.

[115] J. Rahmer, P. Börnert, J. Groen, C. Bos, "Three-dimensional radial ultrashort echo-time imaging with T2 adapted sampling", *Magn Reson Med*, vol. 55, pp. 1075–1082, 2006.

[116] G. Bydder, J. Pennock, R. Steiner, S. Khenia, J. Payne, I. Young, "The short TI inversion recovery sequence – an approach to MR imaging of the abdomen", *Magn Reson Med*, vol. 3, pp. 251–254, 1985.

[117] D. Peters, F. Korosec, T. Grist, W. Block, K. Vigen, J. Holden, C. Mistretta, "Undersampled projection reconstruction applied to MR angiography", *Magn Reson Med*, vol. 43, pp. 91–101, 2000.

[118] T. Gu, F. Korosec, W. Block, S. Fain, Q. Turk, D. Lum, Y. Zhou, T. Grist, V. Haughton, C. Mistretta, "PC VIPR: a high-speed 3D phase-contrast method for flow quantification and high-resolution angiography", *AJNR Am J Neuroradiol.*, vol. 26, pp. 743–749, 2005.

[119] S. Winkelmann, T. Schaeffter, T. Koehler, H. Eggers, O. Doessel, "An Optimal Radial Profile Order Based on the Golden Ratio for Time-Resolved MRI", *IEEE Trand Med Imaging*, vol. 26, pp. 68–76, 2007.

[120] M. Livio, *The Golden Ratio: The story of Phi, The Worlds's most astonishing number*, Broadway Books, New York, 2002.

[121] P. Anderson, "Linear pixel shuffling for image processing: an introduction", *J Electron Imaging*, vol. 2, pp. 147–154, 1993.

[122] J. Rahmer, J. Keupp, S. Caruthers, "Self-Navigated Motion Compensation in Simultaneous 19F/1H 3D Radial Imaging using Golden Means Profile Interleaving", in *Proceedings of the 16th Annual Meeting of ISMRM*, Toronto, Canada, p. 1471, 2008.

[123] R. Chan, E. Ramsay, C. Cunningham, D. Plewes, "Temporal Stability of Adaptive 3D Radial MRI Using Multidimensional Golden Means", *Magn Reson Med*, vol. 61, pp. 354–363, 2009.

[124] V. Rasche, D. Holz, R. Proksa, "MR fluoroscopy using projection reconstruction multi-gradient-echo (prMGE) MRI", *Magn Reson Med*, vol. 42, pp. 324–334, 1999.

[125] P. Kellman, F. Epstein, E. McVeigh, "Adaptive sensitivity encoding incorporating temporal filtering (TSENSE)", *Magn Reson Med*, vol. 45, pp. 846–852, 2001.

[126] P. Gatehouse & G. Bydder, "Magnetic resonance imaging of short T2 components in tissue", *Clin Radiol*, vol. 58, pp. 1–19, 2003.

[127] M. Robson, P. Gatehouse, M. Bydder, G. Bydder, "Magnetic resonance: an introduction to ultrashort TE (UTE) imaging", *J Comput Assist Tomogr*, vol. 27, pp. 825–846, 2003.

[128] P. Bottomley, C. Hardy, R. Argersinger, G. Allen-Moore, "A review of 1H NMR relaxation in pathology: are T1 and T2 diagnostic?", *Med Phys*, vol. 14, pp. 1–37, 1987.

[129] J. B. M. Warntjes, O. Dahlqvist Leinhard, J. West, P. Lundberg, "Rapid Magnetic Resonance Quantification on the Brain: Optimization for Clinical Usage", *Magn Reson Med*, vol. 60, pp. 320–329, 2008.

[130] M. Lansberg, V. Thijs, M. O'Brien, J. Ali, A. de Crespigny, D. Tong, M. Moseley, G. Albers, "Evolution of apparent diffusion coefficient, diffusion-weighted, and T2-weighted signal intensity of acute stroke", *AJNR Am J Neuroradiol*, vol. 22, pp. 637–44, 2001.

[131] P. Tofts, *Quantitative MRI of the brain*, John Wiley & Sons, 2003.

[132] A. Crawley & R. Henkelman, "A comparison of One-Shot and Recovery Methods in T1 imaging", *Magn Reson Med*, vol. 7, pp. 23–34, 1988.

[133] I. Kay & R. Henkelman, "Practical Implementation and Optimization of One-Shot T1 Imaging", *Magn Reson Med*, vol. 22, pp. 414–424, 1991.

[134] A. Fischer, F. Breuer, M. Blaimer, N. Seiberlich, P. Jakob, "Accelerated Dynamic Imaging by Reconstructing Sparse Differences Using Compressed Sensing", in *Proceedings of the 16th Annual Meeting of ISMRM*, Toronto, Canada, p. 341, 2008.

[135] H. Jung, J. Ye, E. Kim, "Improved k-t BLAST and k-t SENSE using FOCUSS", *Phys Med Biol*, vol. 52, pp. 3201–3226, 2007.

[136] R. Duda, P. Hart, D. Stork, *Pattern Classification*, 2 ed., Wiley, New York, 2001.

[137] M. Aharon, M. Elad, A. Bruckstein, "K-SVD: An algorithm for designing overcomplete dictionaries for sparse representation", *IEEE Trans Signal Process*, vol. 54, pp. 4311–4322, 2006.

[138] G. Wright, "Magnetic resonance imaging", *IEEE Signal Processing Magazine*, vol. 14, pp. 56–66, 1977.

[139] V. Olafsson, D. Noll, J. Fessler, "Fast joint reconstruction of dynamic R2* and field maps in functional MRI", *IEEE Trans Med Imaging*, vol. 27, pp. 1177–88, 2008.

[140] R. Kroeker & R. Henkelman, "Analysis of biological NMR relaxation data with continuous distributions of relaxation times", *J Magn Reson*, vol. 69, pp. 218–235, 1986.

[141] S. Kolind, C. Laule, I. Vavasour, D. Li, A. Traboulsee, B. Madler, G. Moore, A. Mackay, "Complementary information from multi-exponential T2 relaxation and diffusion tensor imaging reveals differences between multiple sclerosis lesions", *Neuroimage*, vol. 40, pp. 77–85, 2008.

[142] A. English, K. Whittall, M. Joy, R. Henkelman, "Quantitative twodimensional time correlation relaxometry", *Magn Reson Med*, vol. 22, pp. 425–434, 1991.

[143] S. Graham, S. Ness, B. Hamilton, M. Bronskill, "Magnetic resonance properties of ex vivo breast tissue at 1.5 T", *Magn Reson Med*, vol. 38, pp. 669–677, 1997.

[144] G. Stanisz & R. Henkelman, "Diffusional anisotropy of T2 components in bovine optic nerve", *Magn Reson Med*, vol. 40, pp. 405–410, 1998.

[145] S. Peled, D. Cory, S. Raymond, D. Kirschner, F. Jolesz, "Water diffusion, T2, and compartmentation in frog sciatic nerve", *Magn Reson Med*, vol. 42, pp. 911–918, 1999.

[146] D. Reiter, P. Lin, K. Fishbein, R. Spencer, "Multicomponent T2 Relaxation Analysis in Cartilage", *Magn Reson Med*, vol. 61, pp. 803–809, 2009.

[147] A. Haase, J. Frahm, W. Hänicke, D. Matthaei, "^{1}H NMR chemical shift selective (CHESS) imaging", *Phys Med Biol*, vol. 30, pp. 341–344, 1985.

[148] W. Dixon, "Simple Proton Spectroscopic Imaging", *Radiology*, vol. 153, pp. 189–194, 1984.

[149] R. Sepponen, J. Sipponen, J. Tanttu, "A method for chemical shift imaging: demonstration of bone marrow involvement with proton chemical shift imaging", *J Comput Assist Tomogr*, vol. 8, pp. 585–587, 1984.

[150] G. Glover & E. Schneider, "Three–point Dixon technique for true water/fat decomposition with B0 inhomogeneity correction", *Magn Reson Med*, vol. 18, pp. 371–383, 1991.

[151] J. Ma, S. Singh, A. Kumar, N. Leeds, L. Broemeling, "Method for efficient fast spin echo Dixon imaging", *Magn Reson Med*, vol. 48, pp. 1021–1027, 2002.

[152] S. Reeder, A. Pineda, Z. Wen, A. Shimakawa, H. Yu, J. Brittain, G. Gold, C. Beaulieu, N. Pelc, "Iterative decomposition of water and fat with echo asymmetry and least-squares estimation (IDEAL): application with fast spin-echo imaging", *Magn Reson Med*, vol. 54, pp. 636–644, 2005.

[153] Q. Xiang, "Two-point water-fat imaging with partially-opposed-phase (POP) acquisition: An asymmetric Dixon method", *Magn Reson Med*, vol. 56, pp. 572–584, 2006.

[154] P. Koken, H. Eggers, P. Börnert, "Fast Single Breath-Hold 3D Abdominal Imaging with Water-Fat Separation", in *Proceedings of the 15th Annual Meeting of ISMRM-ESMRMB*, Berlin, Germany, p. 1623, 2007.

[155] H. Yu, A. Shimakawa, C. McKenzie, W. Lu, S. Reeder, S. Hinks, J. Brittain, "Phase and amplitude correction for multi-echo water-fat separation with bipolar acquisitions", *J Magn Reson Imaging*, vol. 31, pp. 1264–1271, 2010.

[156] H. Yu, C. McKenzie, A. Shimakawa, S. Reeder, J. Brittain, "Bipolar Multi-Echo Water-Fat Separation: Phase Correction Using Parallel Imaging", in *Proceedings of the 16th Annual Meeting of ISMRM*, Toronto, Canada, p. 648, 2008.

[157] H. Yu, A. Shimakawa, C. McKenzie, J. Brittain, S. Reeder, "Multiecho Water-Fat Separation and Simultaneous R2* Estimation With Multifrequency Fat Spectrum Modeling", *Magn Reson Med*, vol. 60, pp. 1122–1134, 2008.

[158] J. Ren, I. Dimitrov, A. Sherry, C. Malloy, "Composition of adipose tissue and marrow fat in humans by 1H NMR at 7 Tesla", *J Lipid Res.*, vol. 49, pp. 2055–2062, 2008.

[159] H. Yu, S. Reeder, A. Shimakawa, J. Brittain, N. Pelc, "Field map estimation with a region growing scheme for iterative 3-point water-fat decomposition", *Magn Reson Med*, vol. 54, pp. 1032–1039, 2005.

[160] W. Huh & J. Fessler, "Water-Fat Decomposition With MR Data Based Regularized Estimation In MRI", in *Proceedings of the 17th Annual Meeting of ISMRM*, Honolulu, Hawaii, p. 2846, 2009.

[161] W. Lu & B. Hargreaves, "Multiresolution field map estimation using golden section search for water-fat separation.", *Magn Reson Med*, vol. 60, pp. 236–244, 2008.

[162] M. Jacob & B. Sutton, "Algebraic Decomposition of Fat and Water in MRI", *IEEE Trans Med Imaging*, vol. 28, pp. 173–184, 2009.

[163] D. Hernando, P. Kellman, J. Haldar, Z.-P. Liang, "Robust Water/Fat Separation in the Presence of Large Field Inhomogeneities Using a Graph Cut Algorithm", *Magn Reson Med*, vol. 63, pp. 79–90, 2010.

[164] D. Dunbar & G. Humphreys, "A Spatial Data Structure for Fast Poisson-Disk Sample Generation", in *Proceedings of SIGGRAPH*, pp. 503–508, 2006.

[165] E. Brodsky, J. Holmes, H. Yu, S. Reeder, "Generalized k-space Decomposition with Chemical Shift Correction for Non-Cartesian Water-Fat Imaging", *Magn Reson Med*, vol. 59, pp. 1151–1164, 2008.

[166] R. Henkelman, P. Hardy, J. Bishop, C. Poon, D Plewes, "Why Fat Is Bright in RARE and Fast Spin Echo Imaging", *J Magn Reson Imaging*, vol. 2, pp. 533–540, 1992.

[167] W. Lu, H. Yu, A. Shimakawa, M. Alley, S. Reeder, B. Hargreaves, "Water-Fat Separation with Bipolar Multiecho Sequances.", *Magn Reson Med*, vol. 60, pp. 198–209, 2008.

[168] M. Lustig & J. Pauly, "Compressive Chemical-Shift-Based Rapid Fat/Water Imaging", in *Proceedings of the 17th Annual Meeting of ISMRM*, Honolulu, Hawaii, p. 2646, 2009.

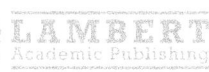

www.ingramcontent.com/pod-product-compliance
Lightning Source LLC
Chambersburg PA
CBHW021109210326
41598CB00017B/1391